Evidence-based Practice for Occupational Therapists

Evidence-based Practice for Occupational Therapists

Second Edition

M Clare Taylor
Principal Lecturer
Department of Occupational Therapy
Coventry University
UK

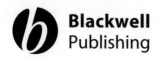

Blackwell
Publishing

© 2000, 2007 Blackwell Publishing Ltd

Editorial offices:
Blackwell Publishing Ltd, 9600 Garsington Road, Oxford OX4 2DQ, UK
Tel: +44 (0)1865 776868
Blackwell Publishing Inc., 350 Main Street, Malden, MA 02148-5020, USA
Tel: +1 781 388 8250
Blackwell Publishing Asia Pty Ltd, 550 Swanston Street, Carlton, Victoria 3053, Australia
Tel: +61 (0)3 8359 1011

First edition published by Blackwell Science Ltd, a Blackwell Publishing Company, 2000
Second edition published 2007 by Blackwell Publishing Ltd, 2007

2   2008

ISBN: 978-1-4051-3700-3

Library of Congress Cataloging-in-Publication Data

Taylor, M. Clare.
    Evidence-based practice for occupational therapists / M. Clare Taylor. – 2nd ed.
        p. ; cm.
    Includes bibliographical references and index.
    ISBN-13: 978-1-4051-3700-3 (pbk. : alk. paper)
    ISBN-10: 1-4051-3700-2 (pbk. : alk. paper)
    1. Occupational therapy.   2. Evidence-based medicine.   I. Title.
        [DNLM: 1. Occupational Therapy–organization & administration.   2. Evidence-Based Medicine.   WB 555 T244 2007]

    RM735.6.T39 2007
    615.8'515–dc22
                        2007004993

A catalogue record for this title is available from the British Library

Set in 10/12.5pt Palatino
by SNP Best-set Typesetter Ltd., Hong Kong
Printed and bound in Singapore
by COS Printers Pte Ltd

The publisher's policy is to use permanent paper from mills that operate a sustainable forestry policy, and which has been manufactured from pulp processed using acid-free and elementary chlorine-free practices. Furthermore, the publisher ensures that the text paper and cover board used have met acceptable environmental accreditation standards.

For further information on Blackwell Publishing, visit our website:
www.blackwellpublishing.com/ot

Dedication

To the memory of my parents, Charles and Audrey Taylor

Contents

Preface   *ix*
Acknowledgements   *xi*

1   Introduction   1

2   Finding the evidence   20

3   Using clinical trials as evidence   43

4   Systematic reviews   66

5   Qualitative research as evidence   86

6   Evidence from other sources   105

7   Making evidence-based practice work   127

8   Carrying out a review of the evidence   145

9   Developing and using guidelines for practice   156

10   Useful resources   168

Glossary   *185*
References   *192*
Index   *205*

Preface

Evidence-based practice (EBP) was often described as the 'buzz phrase' of the 1990s, implying that it was a fad or a fashionable trend. Unlike other fads, EBP did not fade away and go out of fashion; it grew and became a global movement. EBP has also evolved. Having begun as a movement within medicine (evidence-based medicine), EBP was adopted as an approach to healthcare. Subsequently it has been adopted by a variety of health and social care professions, including occupational therapy. Each profession has attempted to make EBP its own. This has required redefinition and refocusing of EBP and, for occupational therapy, the formulation of a definition of evidence-based occupational therapy (EBOT). The advance of an evidence-based approach to social care has led to the elaboration of different approaches to the nature of evidence. All of these developments have been acknowledged within this second edition of the book.

The first edition tended to concentrate on the basic skills of EBP. Whilst this emphasis is still important, there is now a need to explore the implementation and development of an evidence-based culture within occupational therapy departments. The chapter on implementing evidence-based practice (Chapter 7) has been enhanced by a discussion of the use of change management to nurture an evidence-based culture. Part of this culture is the development, by groups of occupational therapists, of guidelines for practice, and this aspect is recognized in a new chapter on 'Developing and using guidelines for practice'.

This book is aimed primarily at undergraduate (pre-registration) occupational therapy students. The nature of occupational therapy education, particularly in the UK, has changed with the introduction of more stringent ethical research procedures as part of the research governance agenda. This has shifted the focus more to literature-based projects than research-based projects for student dissertations. Chapter 8 ('Carrying out a review of the evidence') is intended to support this shift.

The aim of all of the reviewing and reworking has been to provide a text that helps on the journey to becoming an evidence-based occupational therapist. I trust that you will find it useful, and I welcome any feedback or comments.

Clare Taylor
December 2006

Acknowledgements

A number of people have helped with the evolution and writing of this book. Particular recognition and thanks are due to Dr Elizabeth Burrows, for propelling me in the direction of evidence-based practice in the first place; to my colleagues and friends within the Department of Occupational Therapy at Coventry University, for their critical proofreading and for providing the ideas for some of the scenarios used in the book; to occupational therapy students and friends around the world, who have shared my journey of development as an evidence-based occupational therapist, and to Pam, for support in all I do.

1: Introduction

'Evidence-based practice' (EBP) was one of the buzzwords (or buzz terms) of health and social care practice in the 1990s (Taylor 2000). However, unlike other trends or fashions, EBP has not gone away; in fact it has become embedded within the fabric and regulation of professional practice. But what *is* evidence-based practice, where did the term come from and how can it help the overworked occupational therapist to make decisions about the effectiveness of her or his practice? This chapter will attempt to answer these questions.

The chapter begins by defining the term 'evidence-based practice' and then outlines the background to, and the need for, an evidence-based approach to occupational therapy (OT) practice. There is often confusion over what is 'research', what is 'audit' and what is 'evidence-based practice'. This chapter will attempt to clarify the differences between these three approaches to finding and using information to improve practice. Having established what evidence-based practice is, and what it is not, the chapter will then outline the process; in other words, how to implement EBP. The nature of evidence will be explored and the debates about types and levels of evidence within health and social care practice will be outlined. The chapter will conclude with an overview of how to use this book as a practical guide to evidence-based practice.

What is evidence-based practice?

The term 'evidence-based *medicine*' was coined at McMaster University medical school in the 1980s as a way of describing a process of problem-based clinical teaching and learning that involved students and clinicians in searching for and evaluating the evidence for clinical practice (Bennett *et al.* 1987; Shin *et al.* 1993). Its philosophical origins, however, can be found in mid-nineteenth-century Paris (Sackett *et al.* 1996), where Pierre Charles Alexandre Louis used statistical analysis to demonstrate that blood letting had no value as a clinical intervention. A key impetus to the development of evidence-based medicine was the work of Archie Cochrane, an epidemiologist, who championed the use of the randomized controlled trial (RCT) (see Chapter 3 for more on RCTs) and systematic reviews (see

Chapter 4) as tools for ensuring that interventions were both effective and efficient (Cochrane 1972).

Sackett *et al.* (1996, p. 71) have defined evidence-based medicine as:

> the conscientious, explicit and judicious use of current best evidence in making decisions about the care of individual patients.

Although 'evidence-based *medicine*' is still a commonly used term, the evidence-based process has broadened and evolved and now 'evidence-based *practice*' is seen as a more appropriate term. The complexity of evidence-based practice and the blending of both the art and sciences of practice within the decision-making process is demonstrated by use of the term 'evidence-informed practice' (Atherton *et al.* 2005), which highlights the need for decision-making to be informed by, but not dominated by, evidence.

The concern most frequently expressed about evidence-based practice is that it will become prescriptive and will lead to cost cutting and 'cook-book' practice (Sackett *et al.* 1996), where there is one recognized, cheap intervention for a specific problem. In OT this would mean a return to the days of *Refer to Occupational Therapy* (Shopland *et al.* 1975), that neat, pocket-sized book that listed all the things the basic grade OT needed to know in order to be able to treat any stroke, head injury, total hip, etc. and remove the need for thinking or clinical reasoning on the part of the OT. Sackett *et al.* (1996) argue strongly that evidence-based practice is only a part of the clinical decision-making process and that any judgments and clinical decisions are based on a mix of clinical expertise and the best available evidence. The aim is to ensure that the interventions used are the most effective and the safest options. External evidence is just one strand of the process and must be blended with clinical judgment and patient preference.

The essence of evidence-based practice is that the decision process is explicit and therefore clearly articulated so that decisions can be explained to the patient/client and justified to colleagues and managers. Evidence is gathered conscientiously but it is used judiciously so that the experience of the OT, the needs of the patient/client, the demands of the system and the up-to-date best evidence are weighed together so that the best care is given. Evidence-based practice should be viewed as a way of thinking critically about every intervention and action and, as such, is just one of the tools of clinical reasoning and reflective practice. However, because of the use of up-to-date best evidence, evidence-based practice is a powerful tool.

The background to evidence-based practice

Gray (2001) proposes that the management of healthcare over the last three decades has developed from the principles of efficiency and quality. Efficiency can be translated into 'doing things cheaply', whilst quality can be translated as 'doing things better'. This has led to a management philosophy of 'doing things right'. This, however, has not always meant using the 'right' or the 'best' intervention. This may sometimes conflict with the health and social care practitioner's philosophy of doing the right thing, in other words doing 'good' instead of 'harm'. Whilst health and social care practice has attempted to do 'good' and the 'right' thing it has not always been possible to argue that the 'right' intervention is based on anything other than common sense. Cochrane (1972) highlighted medicine's collective ignorance on the effects and effectiveness of healthcare. He proposed that less than 15% of all medical interventions were based on clear clinical trials of effectiveness.

Gray (2001) argues that the philosophy of healthcare management for the twenty-first century will be 'doing the right things right' and that this will mean making decisions about interventions that are based on good evidence and that may have a profound effect on the nature of clinical practice. Research and practice need to be drawn together so that practice is underpinned by sound evidence, and so that clinicians can demonstrate to service managers that they are 'doing the right things right' (Gray 2001, p. 20). The problem for occupational therapists, very often, is defining and measuring what 'good' and 'sound' evidence actually means.

The development of evidence-based OT

The medical roots and philosophy of evidence-based practice might appear to sit uncomfortably with the growing acceptance of the social model philosophy within OT and the focus on a client-centred model of practice. However, evidence-based practice has been explored and discussed in the OT literature for some time, with special issues of various OT journals dedicated to EBP (e.g. *British Journal of Occupational Therapy* 1997, 2001; *Canadian Journal of Occupational Therapy* 1998; see Further reading), books (e.g. Taylor 2000; Law 2002) and articles on implementing EBP (e.g. Brown & Rodgers 1999). A note of caution has been raised by Blair and Robertson (2005, p. 272), who argue that OT has adopted 'a predominantly pragmatic and acquiescent approach' and needs to have a more thoughtful and critical understanding of the philosophy and implications of a truly evidence-based approach to practice.

As Dubouloz *et al.* (1999) pointed out, occupational therapists have been slow to integrate research evidence into their clinical decision-making processes. Client-centred evidence and research evidence were seen as incompatible. In order to recognize the range of evidence available to the occupational therapist, evidence-based OT has been defined as:

> Client-centred enablement of occupation, based on client information and a critical review of relevant research, expert consensus and past experience
> (Canadian Association of Occupational Therapists *et al.* 1999, p. 267).

Whilst the Canadian definition of evidence-based OT highlights the breadth of evidence available to us, Cusick (2001, p. 103) argued that evidence-based OT was more than using a range of evidence to ensure that interventions are effective. She argued that evidence-based OT was about 'asking the right questions':

> When we practice with evidence, it means we should ask ourselves the following question: 'am I doing the right thing in the right way with the right person at the right time in the right place for the right result – and am I the right person to be doing it?'

These are challenging questions, which will make us look at all aspects of our practice in a new and critical light; we will need the courage to change practices that are shown to be ineffective or even harmful. EBP will, however, also give us the tools to ensure that OT practice is seen as effective and valuable within the current political climate.

Thus, evidence-based OT is a way of thinking critically about all aspects of OT interventions and using the breadth of potential sources of 'evidence' conscientiously, judiciously, explicitly *and* critically, within a framework of reflection and clinical reasoning.

Whilst the main focus of this book is the use and critical appraisal of the research evidence, the other sources of evidence will not be ignored as we explore the skills and activities that can enable us to become evidence-based occupational therapists.

Comparison of research, audit and evidence-based practice

The terms 'research', 'audit' and 'evidence-based practice' are liberally used within the healthcare literature, but how well do practitioners understand exactly what the different terms mean? This section will attempt to tease out the differences and similarities between research, audit and evidence-based practice.

Defining the terms

'Research' has been defined as:

> a systematic process of gathering and synthesising empirical data so as to generate knowledge about a given population for a selected topic
>
> (Bailey 1991, p. 1).

Whilst 'audit' has been defined as:

> the systematic critical analysis of the quality of medical care, including the procedures used in diagnosis and treatment, the use of resources and the resulting outcome and quality of life for the patient
>
> (Sale 1996, p. 71).

Finally, as stated earlier, 'evidence-based practice' has been defined as:

> the conscientious, explicit and judicious use of current best evidence in making decisions about the care of individuals
>
> (Sackett *et al*. 1996, p. 71).

Similarities and differences

There are many similarities between research, audit and evidence-based practice. There are also some crucial differences. These are summarized in Table 1.1.

Research, audit and evidence-based practice are all *systematic* processes for finding information to improve and refine interventions and practice. But, whilst research aims to generate new knowledge, both audit and evidence-based practice use existing practice and existing knowledge to review and improve interventions.

The outcomes of research may change practice throughout the world. The outcomes of audit may change practice within one particular setting. The outcomes of evidence-based practice may influence the interventions used with one person, within one department, or at a regional or national level if clinical guidelines are developed.

Research is about generating evidence, audit is about assessing practice, and evidence-based practice is about putting evidence into current practice. As already mentioned, Gray (2001, p. 20) talks about evidence-based practice as 'doing the right things right'. Research is used to tell us what the right things are; audit tells us if we are doing those things right; and evidence-based practice draws these two strands together to help the clinician to use the right intervention properly.

The OT process is essentially the same as the processes of research, audit and evidence-based practice in that a problem needs to be identified, an intervention must be planned and carried out, and the outcome must be assessed and evaluated.

Table 1.1 Similarities and differences of research, audit and evidence-based practice.

Research	Audit	Evidence-based practice
Systematic investigation to increase the sum of knowledge	Systematic approach to identify possible improvements and mechanisms to bring them about	Systematic review of evidence to guide clinical interventions
Aims to identify the most effective form of treatment	Aims to compare actual performance against agreed standards of practice	Aims to use evidence to underpin clinical decision-making
Results extend to the general population	Results apply only to the population examined	Results apply to a particular problem, intervention and outcome
May be a one-off study	The process is ongoing and continuous	Provides a philosophy for decision-making
Data collection is complex, with new data being collected	Data collection is via records and follow-up of patients	Data are drawn from existing research and other sources

The need for an evidence-based approach to practice

As occupational therapists, in order to survive in the current health and social care climate, we need to demonstrate that our interventions are effective both clinically and economically. But where do we find the evidence to support our claims to clinical effectiveness and cost effectiveness? As Table 1.2 illustrates, the range of published literature available that *might* contain the evidence for practice is vast and ever growing.

This list is by no means exhaustive. Nor does it include what is known as 'grey' literature. The 'grey' literature is literature that has been published or is in the public domain that lacks an ISBN (International Standard Book Number) in the case of a book or an International Standard Serial Number (ISSN) in the case of a serial publication such as a journal. This means, therefore, that the grey literature is not easily accessed from databases. Grey literature includes theses and dissertations, which are held in university and departmental libraries; conference presentations and proceedings, which may not be fully reported; and all manner of other material on research and projects that has been written up but goes no further than a library shelf. As well as the grey literature the web also gives access to a vast amount of literature, some of which will be useful evidence whilst some will reflect one person's opinion (Chapter 6 will explore the value of the web for the evidence-based OT). Occupational therapists in the UK are now being educated at degree level, with a growing number undertaking postgraduate studies. They are all spending long hours researching and writing dissertations and yet few of these will be published or become available to a wider audience. Many of these, on well-worn topics, may not be of great value to a wider audience, such as:

■ how nurses/doctors/GPs/the multidisciplinary team (MDT) view the role of OT;
■ the role of OT within mental health.

Others, though, provide useful evidence and deserve to be available to a wider audience; for example:

■ homophobia amongst OT students: issues, incidence and implications (Haddon-Silver 1993);
■ does the Rivermead Extended ADL Score indicate a patient's level of independence after discharge? (Cooper 1995);
■ do OT students consider sexual orientation when implementing treatment? (Littlewood 1997);
■ an audit of the reliability of the Frenchay Activities Index (Piercy 1998).

The College of Occupational Therapists' (COT) library holds copies of many masters and doctoral theses produced by occupational therapists. However, too much valuable OT evidence remains as grey literature and, as such, is unavailable to the occupational therapist who wishes to become more evidence-based and might be struggling to find relevant research evidence within their practice area.

Table 1.2 Journals with the potential for providing the evidence base for OT interventions.

Access by Design
American Journal of Occupational Therapy
American Journal of Physical Medicine and Rehabilitation
American Rehabilitation
Archives of Physical Medicine and Rehabilitation
Australian Occupational Therapy Journal
British Journal of Learning Disabilities
British Journal of Occupational Therapy
Canadian Journal of Occupational Therapy
Clinical Rehabilitation
Disability and Rehabilitation
Disability and Society
Evidence-based Mental Health
Health Service Journal
International Journal of Rehabilitation Research
Irish Occupational Therapy Journal
International Journal of Therapy and Rehabilitation
Israeli Journal of Occupational Therapy
Journal of Allied Health
Journal of Applied Research in Intellectual Abilities
Journal of Evaluation in Clinical Practice
Journal of Hand Therapy
Journal of Head Trauma Rehabilitation
Journal of Interprofessional Care
Journal of Occupational Science: Australia
Journal of Rehabilitation
Journal of Rehabilitation Research and Development
Neuropsychology Rehabilitation
New Zealand Journal of Occupational Therapy
Occupational Therapy in Health Care
Occupational Therapy in Mental Health
Occupational Therapy International
Occupational Therapy Journal of Research: Participation, Occupation and Health
Occupational Therapy News
Occupational Therapy Practice
Physical and Occupational Therapy in Geriatrics
Physical and Occupational Therapy in Pediatrics
Scandinavian Journal of Occupational Therapy
Scandinavian Journal of Rehabilitation Medicine
Social Science and Medicine
South African Journal of Occupational Therapy

Busy occupational therapists cannot hope to keep up to date with all the possible sources of evidence, nor can they read and critically appraise all of the articles relevant to their practice. This is why an evidence-based approach to practice is needed. Evidence-based practice provides occupational therapists with a systematic framework for reviewing the evidence to underpin their practice. Sackett (1997) has shown that in the majority of cases an evidence-based approach does not, in fact, change the intervention decision. What evidence-based practice does, however, is give occupational therapists the tools and the evidence to justify that intervention to themselves, the patient/client and the management.

The process of evidence-based practice

Evidence-based practice is a process, which is essentially the same as both the research process and the OT process. All of these processes are based on a number of stages, which include:

- identify a problem;
- plan/design an intervention/action;
- carry out the intervention/action;
- evaluate the process and the outcome.

Rosenberg and Donald (1995) have identified four stages in the evidence-based practice process:

- formulate a clear clinical question based on the patient's problem;
- search the literature for relevant clinical articles/evidence;
- evaluate (critically appraise) this evidence for its validity and usefulness;
- implement useful findings in clinical practice.

Sackett *et al.* (2000) added a fifth and final stage:

- evaluate the outcome.

Having established what the patient's/client's problems are, evidence-based practice can be initiated by asking 'clinical' questions related to diagnosis, prognosis, treatment, iatrogenic harm, quality of care and health economics (Rosenberg & Donald 1995). The question should focus on the problem, the intervention and the outcome. Evidence-based questions are usually articulated in terms of:

What is the evidence for the effectiveness of x (the intervention) for y (the outcome) in a patient with z (the problem or diagnosis)?

This might fit very nicely into medical practice when thinking about whether treatment with aspirin and warfarin will reduce the risk of stroke in an elderly lady with hypertension, but how can it relate to the complexities of OT practice?

Herbert *et al.* (2005, p. 12) expand the notion of the clinical question to include:

- effects of intervention;
- patients' experiences;
- the course of the condition, or life-course (prognosis);
- the accuracy of diagnostic tests or assessments.

Whilst broadening the idea of the clinical question beyond assessing the potential effectiveness of an intervention, this approach still does not address the totality of OT practice. However, with the basic OT skills of creative thinking, it is perfectly possible to focus on a problem, an intervention and an outcome and thus initiate evidence-based practice.

If we adopt Cusick's (2001) approach of asking the right questions, we can utilize an evidence-based approach to all stages of the OT process, for example:

- Are we the right people?
  Should this person have been referred to OT?
- Are we doing the right thing?
  Not only is this the right intervention, but also is this the right assessment tool?
- Are we doing it the right way?
  What is the most effective model or frame of reference?
- Are we doing it with the right clients?
  Do *all* patients/clients with this problem need to be seen by an occupational therapist, or just those with other particular problems?
- Are we doing it at the right time?
  Should I see this client in the morning or the afternoon?
  Should I see them every day or just once a month?
- Is it being done in the right place?
  Would I be better working with this patient/client in their own home rather than in hospital?

Bennett and Bennett (2000) developed a framework for the use of evidence-based practice in OT (see Fig. 1.1). They show evidence-based practice to be an approach that can be used at every stage of the OT process. The search for, and appraisal of, relevant evidence can be used to support the clinical decisions that are made at each stage of the OT process. Bennett and Bennett's framework highlights the importance of both research evidence and evidence drawn from other sources, such as the therapist's experiential evidence and the client's preferences and values.

By blending Cusick's (2001) series of 'right' questions with Bennett and Bennett's (2000) framework we have a clear overview of the ways in which evidence-based practice can be used throughout the OT process to explore and support the effectiveness of our actions and interventions as occupational therapists.

Each stage of the evidence-based practice process will be explored in this book. Asking and formulating a 'clear clinical question from the patient's problem' will be discussed below. The three remaining stages of finding, appraising and using evidence will form the basis of the remaining chapters. The final stage (evaluating the outcome), whilst important, is beyond the scope of this introductory text.

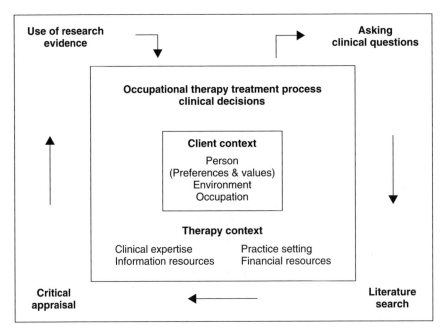

Figure 1.1 Bennett and Bennett's framework for evidence-based occupational therapy. (From Bennett, S. & Bennett, J.W. (2000) The process of evidence-based practice in occupational therapy: informing clinical decisions. *Australian Occupational Therapy Journal* **172**, 171–178. Reproduced with permission from Blackwell Publishing Ltd.)

Asking useful questions

The first stage in the search for evidence to underpin practice is to ask a clear question. This question will be used to guide the search for evidence and so must be clear and specific, otherwise a vast amount of evidence may be found that has little, if any, relevance to the initial question. A great deal of time can be wasted down the interesting side tracks this may produce. However, getting side-tracked will not answer the original question and may reinforce negative assumptions about the value, or lack of value, of an evidence-based approach to practice.

As outlined above, a useful question consists of:

■ a problem;
■ an intervention;
■ an outcome.

In other words, you must identify:

■ 'who' – i.e. a patient or client group with a particular occupational or clinical problem;
■ 'what' – i.e. the intervention/assessment/task you think might be of value for this problem;
■ 'why'– i.e. the outcome or reason for using the intervention/assessment/task.

Without the outcome the question can become vague and woolly and any evidence found will have limited value in answering the question. The more time you spend formulating your question the easier the task of finding the right evidence specific to your needs.

Some authors (Richardson *et al.* 1995) argue that a 'well-built' question should include not just an intervention but also a comparative intervention. This is common practice when looking at treatment interventions within a medical context when the effectiveness of drug A is compared with that of drug B. This comparative approach may have relevance to some evidence-based practitioners in OT; however, for many OT problems comparison of interventions may not be appropriate or useful.

Richardson *et al.* (1995) refer to the elements of the question (the problem, the intervention/comparison, the outcome) as the 'anatomy' of an evidence-based question. As we will see in Chapter 2 (Finding the evidence), the clearer you are about each element of the question and the components of each element, the more successful you will be in finding evidence and answering your question. Table 1.3 outlines the four elements of an evidence-based question.

Practical applications of this process will now be discussed. Scenarios will be used to create evidence-based questions. A flexible approach to the development of evidence-based questions has been adopted, allowing for a range of applications of evidence-based practice to be illustrated. These scenarios and questions will be used in later chapters to illustrate the application of evidence-based practice for OT.

Table 1.3 Elements of a well-built evidence-based question.

Problem	Intervention	Comparative intervention	Outcome
Describe your patient/client/client group and her/his/their problem. This may be a diagnosis, a functional problem or an occupational performance problem. The description should also include all key information, e.g. age, sex, occupational status	Describe the main intervention/ assessment/task	*If applicable* Describe the comparative or alternative intervention/ assessment/task. This may also take the form of alternative approaches to the intervention, e.g. group or individual sessions; different frequency of intervention	Describe what you hope to achieve or what effect the intervention may have on your patient/client/client group

After the scenario is described, the problem, intervention and outcome will be highlighted and an evidence-based question will be developed.

▪ Scenario 1.1 ▪

You have recently been appointed to a post that includes a unit specializing in the care of people who are HIV-positive or who have AIDS. You are exploring potential areas of OT intervention. You notice that many of the clients appear to be experiencing high levels of anxiety, which limits their occupational performance. You have also read that levels of anxiety may affect the body's immune responses. You feel that an area of OT intervention might be in anxiety management. However, before embarking on designing an anxiety management programme you decide to explore whether this is an effective intervention and what evidence exists to support your proposal for establishing anxiety management as part of the OT intervention on the unit.

Problem	Intervention	Outcome
Anxiety in clients with HIV/AIDS	Anxiety management	Improved function and occupational performance; improved immunity; improved quality of life

What is the evidence for the value of anxiety management as a means of improving function/occupational performance/immunity/quality of life in clients who are HIV-positive or who have AIDS?

▪ Scenario 1.2 ▪

You have been running an outpatient group and course on joint protection and energy conservation for clients with rheumatoid arthritis (RA). The energy conservation aspect of the group seems to be particularly successful. You are preparing a proposal to extend the energy conservation group to include other clients who experience periods of fatigue, such as people with multiple sclerosis (MS) or AIDS. You decide to explore the evidence base for using energy conservation education as a way of decreasing fatigue with these client groups. You are also interested to explore whether group or individual sessions are more effective or whether sessions should focus solely on information or should include discussion and a self-help focus.

Problem	Intervention	Alternative interventions	Outcome
Fatigue associated with: ▪ MS ▪ HIV/AIDS ▪ RA	Energy conservation	Individual or group session; length of course; handouts and/or discussion; self-help	Improved quality of life; increased occupational performance; decreased fatigue

What is the evidence for the value of energy conservation as a means of improving quality of life/occupational performance and decreasing levels of fatigue in clients who experience high levels of fatigue associated with chronic illnesses such as MS, AIDS and RA?

▪ Scenario 1.3 ▪

As a final-year OT student you are expected to carry out either a piece of empirical research or a systematic review of the literature pertinent to an area of OT practice. One of your fieldwork placements was spent at a specialist rehabilitation unit for people who have suffered brain injury. Whilst at the unit you noticed that many of the clients had memory impairments. The approach used with these clients was to give each client a variety of memory aids. Working with a number of clients, you had begun to explore alternative approaches such as using activities and groups as well as aids and education to improve memory function. You decide, for your final-year project, to carry out a systematic review of the evidence into the effectiveness of a number of approaches to improving memory function.

Problem	Intervention	Alternative interventions	Outcome
Memory impairment following brain injury	Memory aids	Group or individual sessions; education or activity	Decrease in confusion; increase in memory function; increase in occupational performance

What is the evidence for the value of memory aids as a means of decreasing confusion and improving memory function and occupational performance in clients with memory impairment as a result of brain injury?

These three scenarios are examples of what might be considered the traditional approach to evidence-based questions, with a clear problem, intervention and outcome. However, as the next three scenarios show, evidence-based practice can also be applied to more general topics or as a preparatory tool for developing research questions.

▪ Scenario 1.4 ▪

You are the OT manager for a mental health trust. You are beginning to explore evidence-based practice and are wondering how an evidence-based approach might be applied to your service. Because of economic and service constraints you are reviewing the value and effectiveness of a number of OT interventions and areas of practice. You are particularly concerned about the value of some of the activity groups within the main OT department. Rather than focusing on one particular activity you decide to adopt a broad evidence-based approach. You decide to explore the concept of 'activity' within a specific diagnostic and symptom context. The majority of clients who attend the various activity groups have some level of depression.

Problem	Intervention	Outcome
Depression	Activity, which could be subdivided to include, e.g.: ▪ exercise ▪ creative writing ▪ pottery	Improved mood

What is the evidence for the value of activity as a means of improving mood in clients with depression?

■ Scenario 1.5 ■

Recently you have been running a horticulture group as part of the activity programme for the eating disorders unit you work on. The group has proved to be remarkably successful. You are keen to carry out some research into the value of horticulture as a purposeful activity, but are unsure about how to start this research. As a way of helping to develop your research ideas you decide to carry out an evidence-based review of the value of horticulture as a purposeful activity.

Problem	Intervention	Outcome
Eating disorders: ■ anorexia ■ bulimia	Horticulture	Improve self-esteem: ■ increase confidence in self ■ increase confidence in abilities

What is the evidence for the value of horticulture as a purposeful activity and means of improving self-esteem and confidence in clients with eating disorders?

■ Scenario 1.6 ■

You have been asked to co-facilitate a support group for people who are carers of patients with Alzheimer's disease. You have some ideas about the potential support needs of carers but are unclear about the specific needs of this particular group of carers. You decide to collect evidence from a range of sources to inform your planning for the support group and its activities. You also hope that the evidence will give you ideas about assessing the outcomes and the success of the group.

Problem	Intervention	Outcome
Support needs/issues of people caring for someone with Alzheimer's disease	A range of interventions including: ■ support groups ■ group work ■ self-help ■ educational group	Guidelines for facilitating a support group

What information can be derived from a range of evidence into the support needs of people caring for someone who has Alzheimer's disease, in order to facilitate a support group?

Whilst some of these questions may appear vague, the aim for all of these questions and scenarios is to use them as tools to illustrate the practical application of evidence-based practice for occupational therapists. The scenarios and questions aim to cover a broad spectrum of OT practice. However, the author acknowledges that it is not practical to explore the totality of OT interventions within one small text.

The nature of 'best evidence'

The Sackett *et al.* (1996) definition of evidence-based practice talks about the use of 'best evidence' to support the clinical decision-making process. However, the nature of 'best evidence' is perhaps the most contentious and debated area of evidence-based practice (Sackett & Wennberg 1997). The traditional view, drawn from evidence-based medicine, has been to adopt a rigid approach to evidence founded on a perception of a hierarchy and levels of research evidence. Table 1.4 outlines the hierarchy of evidence. The origin of this hierarchy is in the work of Fletcher and Sackett (Canadian Task Force on the Periodic Health Examination 1979) whilst current discussion of levels of evidence can be found on the Centre for Evidence-based Medicine website (http://www.cebm.net/levels_of_evidence.asp).

However, this approach ignores two major factors. The first is that there is a breadth of potential research approaches, which might be appropriately viewed as 'best evidence'. The second is that many definitions of evidence-based practice include not only research but also the therapist's experiential knowledge and the client's perspective as potential sources of evidence.

The potential range of research approaches and types that might be seen as evidence includes:

- randomized controlled trials (RCTs);
- systematic reviews of RCTs;
- controlled clinical trials;
- nonrandomized experimental studies;
- single-case design studies
- cohort studies;
- cross-sectional studies;
- longitudinal studies;
- correlational studies;
- qualitative research studies;
- systematic reviews of qualitative research;
- surveys;
- delphi studies;
- consensus studies;
- case studies.

The question for the evidence-based occupational therapist is, which of this long list might be the 'best evidence' for me to use to address my particular evidence-based question? As Sackett (1998) and Sackett and Wennberg (1997) argue, the

Table 1.4 Levels of evidence.

Systematic reviews and meta-analyses of randomized controlled trials
Randomized controlled trials
Nonrandomized experimental studies
Nonexperimental studies
Descriptive studies
Respected opinion, expert discussion

nature of the 'best evidence' depends upon the type of evidence-based question being asked. Table 1.5 gives an overview of the types of research evidence that might be appropriate for the different types of evidence-based question.

Having established a list of the potential types of research evidence to address a particular question, the evidence-based occupational therapist's next task is to decide whether there is a particular order of hierarchy of the types of evidence, to ensure that the 'best' evidence is found.

Developing a hierarchy of the most appropriate evidence for the effectiveness of interventions is relatively straightforward. The hierarchy outlined in Table 1.4 was developed to show the value and weighting of evidence for the effectiveness of interventions, with systematic reviews of RCTs seen as the most rigorous and reliable form of evidence. The Centre for Evidence-based Medicine (CEBM) has developed similar hierarchies for the following (Phillips *et al.* 2001):

■ therapy/prevention/aetiology/harm questions;
■ prognosis questions;
■ diagnosis questions;
■ differential diagnosis/symptoms questions;
■ economic questions.

The appropriateness and value of a similar hierarchy for qualitative research is much more questionable, with many authors (e.g. Barbour 2001; Pawson *et al.* 2003) arguing that, whilst it might be possible critically to appraise the rigour and strength of a particular qualitative study it is neither possible nor appropriate to locate different types of qualitative studies and approaches within a hierarchy.

Table 1.5 Appropriate research evidence for particular types of evidence-based questions.

Effectiveness of interventions
Systematic reviews of RCTs
RCTs
Other experimental designs, e.g. controlled clinical trials
Single subject design studies

Client's experiences and perceptions
Qualitative research studies
Descriptive research studies, e.g. surveys
Systematic reviews of qualitative research

Appropriateness of assessments
Cross-sectional studies
Measurement studies

Prognosis and life-course
Cohort studies
Longitudinal studies
Correlational studies

Developing a hierarchy of potential evidence should help to narrow the focus of the search to a specific type of research evidence that will address the particular evidence-based question (the topic of searching is dealt with in Chapter 2). Once a research paper has been found, it may still not provide the 'best' evidence. Deciding whether any research paper is 'best' or 'good' is achieved through critically appraising the quality of the research against a series of questions or criteria (Chapters 3, 4 and 5 deal with the critical appraisal of the main types of research evidence).

The identification of the 'best' evidence is a complex task. The potential range of evidence is broad and should not solely focus on research evidence. Using specific types of research evidence to address particular evidence-based questions may seem the most useful approach. However, it may also act as a constraint, if not a straightjacket, to the development of a broad perspective on the 'best evidence' with which to answer evidence-based questions. Certainly an RCT or a systematic review should provide powerful evidence for the effectiveness of a particular intervention; it should not, however, be the only evidence required for clinical reasoning and decision-making. Pawson *et al.* (2003) argue, from a social care perspective, that evidence should include:

■ organizational knowledge
■ practitioner knowledge
■ user knowledge
■ research knowledge
■ policy knowledge

thus acknowledging the breadth and complexity of evidence to be considered, especially within a social care context.

Evidence from research studies can only give a partial answer to any evidence-based question. The research evidence must be balanced with information from the client about their values and perspectives, as well as the therapist's experiential knowledge. The intervention or action decision will also be influenced by contextual factors such as service priorities and resources, as well as local and national policies. Evidence should not be seen in terms of a hierarchy but in terms of pieces of a complex jigsaw, which together provide the 'best evidence' to answer any evidence-based question. Figure 1.2 attempts to draw together the threads that underpin the decision-making process that focuses on any particular evidence-based question.

How to use this book

The main aim of this book is to make evidence-based practice accessible to occupational therapists. The scenarios and questions outlined in this chapter will be used later in the book as practical illustrations of finding, appraising and using evidence to review the effectiveness of OT interventions and practice. Each chapter will also include activities to help you consolidate your evidence-based practice skills.

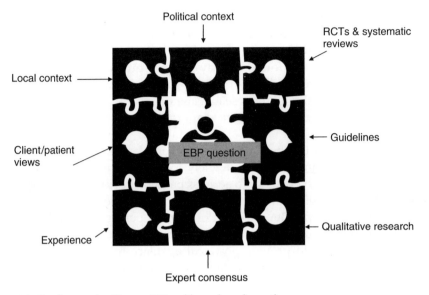

Figure 1.2 The jigsaw of evidence. EBP, evidence-based practice.

The book will explore each stage of the evidence-based practice process in turn – beginning with finding the evidence, then looking at appraising various types of research evidence (RCTs, systematic reviews, qualitative research and other types of evidence) before considering how evidence-based practice might work in OT practice settings. The book concludes by giving an annotated listing of a variety of resources that might be helpful to the evidence-based practitioner. Whilst the flow of the book follows the stages of the evidence-based practice process, it is the author's intention that each chapter can stand alone and can be read separately. It is not the author's intention that the reader starts at page 1 and reads studiously and conscientiously to the end of the book. However, it is the author's intention that, when you finish working through this book, you should have a clear and practical grasp of how an evidence-based approach can help occupational therapists to explore and evaluate the effectiveness of their practice.

▨ ▨

Activity

- Think of a client/patient or scenario from your practice.
- Look at the client/scenario in terms of the elements of evidence-based practice:
  - problem;
  - intervention/alternative intervention;
  - outcome(s).
- Outline the components of each of these elements for your client/scenario.
- Write an evidence-based question, using the elements you have identified.

▨ ▨

Further reading

The following references will be useful for the reader who wishes to explore the background to evidence-based practice further, or who wishes to explore wider issues within the remit of evidence-based practice.

American Occupational Therapy Association (1999 onwards) *American Occupational Therapy Journal* **53**(5 onwards) [Since 1999 the AOTA has published an 'Evidence-based Practice Forum' to explore and convey information about the nature and process of evidence-based practice within occupational therapy.]

British Journal of Therapy and Rehabilitation (1996) Supplement on evidence-based practice and mental health. *British Journal of Therapy and Rehabilitation* **3**(12), 659–670.

Canadian Association of Occupational Therapists (1998) Special edition on evidence-based practice. *Canadian Journal of Occupational Therapy* **65**(3).

College of Occupational Therapists (1997) Special edition on evidence-based practice. *British Journal of Occupational Therapy* **60**(11).

Gray, J.A.M. (2001) *Evidence-based Healthcare,* 2nd edn. Edinburgh: Churchill Livingstone.

Hope, T. (1997) *Evidence-based Patient Choice.* London: King's Fund.

Rosenberg, W. & Donald, A. (1995) Evidence based medicine: an approach to clinical problem-solving. *British Medical Journal* **310**, 1122–1126.

Sackett, D.L., Rosenberg, W.M.C., Gray, J.A.M., Haynes, R.B. & Richardson, W.S. (1996) Evidence-based medicine: what it is and what it isn't. *British Medical Journal* **312**, 71–72.

Straus, S., Richardson, W.S., Glasziou, P. & Haynes, R.B. (2005) *Evidence-based Medicine: How to Practice and Teach EBM,* 3rd edn. Edinburgh: Elsevier Churchill Livingstone.

Trinder, L. & Reynolds, S. (eds) (2000) *Evidence-based Practice: A Critical Appraisal.* Oxford: Blackwell Science.

2: Finding the evidence

Having decided to adopt an evidence-based approach to practice and having developed an evidence-based question, the next stage in the process is to attempt to find the evidence. Having found the evidence you will need to appraise it; this will be considered in Chapters 3 to 5. This chapter will concentrate on the process of searching for and finding the evidence. The chapter will begin by reviewing the potential sources of evidence that are available to the evidence-based practitioner. The process of searching will then be outlined and the scenarios and problems developed in the previous chapter will be used to illustrate the successes and pitfalls of searching. The various searches will also use a variety of databases and sources of material to allow the reader to compare the potential usefulness of a range of resources. Having found the references and citations of evidence it is important to be able to access and acquire the material. The chapter will conclude by discussing ways of accessing and then storing evidence. The chapter will also include a number of activities for the reader to consolidate her or his evidence-based skills.

Sources of evidence

We noted in Chapter 1 that there are a variety of potential sources of evidence for the evidence-based practitioner, and that different types of research may be more appropriate for particular evidence-based questions.

The next question to ask is where can the evidence-based occupational therapist find this evidence? Research information can be found in conference proceedings, books and journals. But which of these will provide the 'best' and most up-to-date information?

Books, conferences or journals?

Common sense might lead us to think that conferences would be the best sources of good-quality, up-to-date research evidence. However, this is not necessarily the case. Conferences are certainly sources of up-to-date and current evidence.

Presenters will often be talking about work still in progress or recently completed. However, conferences will not always be the source of the best-quality information. Conference presentations are usually subject to relatively low-level quality filters. The conference committee will review and choose papers for presentation based on a number of criteria. One of these criteria may be the rigour of the research, but other factors will also influence decisions about inclusion of papers. Conferences and conference proceedings should be viewed as useful sources of contacts with experts and ideas about current developments in the field but should not be seen as sources of high-quality evidence.

Books should also be viewed with caution. The major problem with books is that they are dated almost as soon as they are published. The process of getting a book from idea to print can take at least two years, by which time knowledge may have moved on. A frequently cited example from the world of evidence-based *medicine* is the evidence for the use of thrombolytic therapy with patients who have had heart attacks. The randomized controlled trial (RCT) evidence was available in 1970 and yet it was not until the late 1980s, some 15–17 years later, that the medical textbooks routinely recommended the use of thrombolytic therapy for patients who had experienced heart attacks (Gray 2001). The evidence might be available, but books may not be the best place to begin a search for *current* best evidence.

The 'best' and most current evidence will be found in journals. However, some journals are 'better' than others. Some journals contain articles that have been rigorously peer reviewed, whilst other journals are less rigorous in their approach. The peer review process attempts to ensure that only good-quality research is published. Reviewers will comment not only on the applicability and readability of the article but also on the rigour of the research design, the robustness of the analysis and the validity of the conclusions being drawn. Journal articles will also include an overview of the methods used in the research and thus allow the reader critically to appraise the quality of the research and its evidence. Journals should provide the major source of good-quality evidence for the evidence-based occupational therapist.

Indexes and databases

Having identified journals as the best sources of evidence, how does the evidence-based occupational therapist find the right articles in the right journals? The novice searcher often goes into a library, finds a likely-looking journal and starts flicking through it in the hope of finding something useful. However, with some 20 occupational therapy (OT)-specific journals and over 20 000 journals published annually (Mulrow 1994), this is not the best approach for the evidence-based occupational therapist. Searching should be systematic and focused.

Bibliographic indexes and databases have been developed to help readers and researchers locate the most suitable information for particular topics.

Databases provide access to information from large numbers of journals (as well as books and conference abstracts, in some cases). Subject headings are used to code and cross-reference each entry. Therefore, by choosing key words the evidence-based occupational therapist can search for the most relevant information for a particular topic or question. Databases are commonly available on-line via the internet, although many will require a password to access them. Chapter 10 contains detailed information on the most appropriate databases for the evidence-based occupational therapist. These databases are listed in Table 2.1.

Specialist evidence-based databases, unlike general databases, employ quality checks, and so will only include citations for work that meets their standards for good evidence.

Databases have different areas of focus. MEDLINE, PubMed and EMBASE have a very medical focus, whilst CINAHL and AMED focus more on allied health. ASSIA, PsychLit and SocioFile draw heavily on social science literature, and ERIC has an educational focus. Thus, some databases will be more suitable for some questions than for others. However, the evidence-based occupational therapist must also be pragmatic. The search for evidence may also be restricted by the local availability of search resources.

Table 2.1 Most relevant databases for the occupational therapist.

General databases
AMED
ASSIA
BIDS
CINAHL
EMBASE
ERIC
MEDLINE
PubMed
PsychLit
SocioFile

OT databases
OTseeker (and its sister physiotherapy database – PEDro)
OTBibSys
OTDBase

Specialist evidence-based databases
Cochrane Library
DARE
Campbell Collaboration
Best Evidence
Clinical Evidence
Health Technology Assessment database

▥ ▥

Activity

▥ Identify what databases are available locally, in:
- hospital and health authority libraries, or other workplace libraries;
- university libraries;
- public libraries.

▥ Identify where you might be able to access and use the internet:
organize passwords for any databases that require them.

▥ ▥

Searching for evidence

The most important things for a successful search are to be organized, systematic and focused. Without these the search will become easily side-tracked into looking at interesting but peripheral (at best) or irrelevant (at worst) areas, or will produce vast amounts of material most of which has limited value in providing an evidence-based answer to the question.

The process of successful searching consists of four stages:

▥ Asking a clear question, identifying the problem, intervention, alternative intervention and outcome (as appropriate).
▥ Identifying the most appropriate library, collection or information source for the question.
▥ Selecting the database most relevant to the question.
▥ Developing a clear search strategy with key words and search terms.

The development of a clear question has been dealt with in the previous chapter. To identify the library or collection that will provide the best information for your question, you need to think:

▥ Whether the search will be done by you or by someone else (e.g. a librarian).
▥ How much time, money and effort you have available and are prepared to spend.
▥ Whether you want immediate access to the literature or are prepared to use Inter-Library Loan to access literature.
▥ Where the focus of the question lies; is it:
- intervention focused;
- focused on a specific diagnosis;
- on management issues;
- on user/client perspectives?

How you answer these will determine your choice of library. It might be that the local Trust libraries have sufficient resources, or you might want to use the College of Occupational Therapists' Library and Information service and resources, or to access a university library. Useful guides to libraries are:

▥ *Guide to Libraries and Information Services in Medicine and Health Care* (Dale 2000)
▥ *ASLIB Directory of Information Sources in the United Kingdom* (Reynard & Reynard 2004)
▥ *Literature Searching: Where to Go and What to Look For* (Chartered Society of Physiotherapy 1996).

To choose the most appropriate database, you need to think:

▥ Whether the focus of the question is medical or broader.
▥ Whether the focus of the search is OT-specific.
▥ Whether the focus of the search will be on British literature or broader.
▥ What types of research are to be accessed, whether the focus is on RCTs or a wider methodological perspective.

The areas of focus of the various databases have already been identified (see also Chapter 10: Useful resources) and must be considered when developing a search strategy. The specialist evidence-based databases (Best Evidence, Cochrane, DARE, OTseeker) will tend to have an RCT focus, whilst other databases will include a wider variety of methodologies.

The final aspect of planning is developing a clear search strategy. This means:

▥ Reviewing the question and identifying key words and terms to be used to drive the search.
▥ Setting limits to the search in terms of language of publication, research design, date of publication.

Most databases do not readily understand 'natural language', the colloquial language we use everyday. However, the majority of databases have a thesaurus of accepted terms and key words. Many medical and medicine-related databases use MeSH terms (medical subject headings). This is a limited list of terms devised by the National Library of Medicine as an indexing tool. MeSH terms are also linked to 'broader', 'narrower' and 'related' terms:

for example, *occupational therapy* can be 'broadened' to either *rehabilitation* or *allied health occupations.*

Related items are indicated by the term 'see':

e.g. *chronic limitation of activity* is related by 'see' to *activities of daily living.*

Most databases have an easily accessible thesaurus to help identify indexing terms.

Most databases use what are known as Boolean operators to help the searcher refine a search question. Thus terms can be combined to focus the search or limits can be set on the search. AND and OR are the key combining terms. Thus a searcher interested in stress management as used by occupational therapists would search using:

STRESS MANAGEMENT **AND** OCCUPATIONAL THERAPY

Whilst another searcher who wanted to make sure she accessed both British and North American literature concerning people with learning disabilities would remember that the Americans use the term 'mental retardation' and so would search with:

LEARNING DISABILITY **OR** MENTAL RETARDATION

to access both sets of literature and terminology. Other Boolean operators include **NOT** – to exclude terms, for example:

ANOREXIA **NOT** BULIMIA

to search for literature about eating disorders but specific to anorexia. The symbol * is used to denote truncate:

e.g. THERAP*

will access citations containing both 'therapy' and 'therapist'.

Many of these areas will be unpacked and explored in the next section, which takes the scenarios and questions developed in the previous chapter and uses them as worked examples of searches.

Examples of searches

The scenarios and questions that were developed in Chapter 1 have been used to form the basis of a number of searches. Each search will be outlined in terms of an overview of the problem, the search terms, the choice of particular databases to be searched, an overview of the searches and a review of the outcomes of the searches.

▪ Scenario 2.1 ▪

Question and search terms

What is the evidence for the value of anxiety management as a means of improving function/ occupational performance/immunity/quality of life in clients who are HIV-positive or who have AIDS?

Problem	Intervention	Outcome
Anxiety in clients with HIV/AIDS	Anxiety management	Improved function and occupational performance; improved immunity; improved quality of life

▪ Search terms 2.1 ▪

Problem	Intervention	Outcome
HIV	anxiety management	activities of daily living
AIDS	stress management	occupational performance
anxiety	rehabilitation	quality of life
		immune response

Choice of databases

Anxiety management, as an intervention, may be carried out by a number of healthcare professionals. Databases that cover a broad healthcare perspective should be used. The focus of the question is on the effectiveness of an intervention; therefore the main source of evidence should be RCTs and systematic reviews of RCTs. The databases chosen for the search were:

▪ CINAHL
▪ OTseeker

This search provided a useful opportunity to compare these two databases (Table 2.2); one is a general healthcare database and the other has a more specific evidence-based OT perspective.

Outcomes of search

The CINAHL search produced a huge number of hits, whereas the OTseeker search produced a much more manageable, and more focused, array of hits. When the output from both searches was compared the CINAHL search gave eight potentially relevant articles, whereas for the OTseeker search all 14 hits were potentially relevant articles and the majority had been given quality scores giving a clear guide as to the potential strength of each article as evidence. However, there were three duplicates within each search. This indicates that the CINAHL search gave little extra information, for this topic. This implies that, for topics covering allied healthcare perspectives, the evidence-based occupational therapist might be best advised to choose OTseeker as the database of choice rather than CINAHL.

Table 2.2 Search strategy: comparing CINAHL and OTseeker.

CINAHL	OTseeker
The search terms: ▪ anxiety ▪ anxiety management ▪ HIV and AIDS ▪ immun* – truncated to access immune, immunity, etc. It was decided to use the terms as natural language rather than via the thesaurus, as this had proved successful in search 2 The various search terms were combined, using AND, with varying degrees of success: ▪ anxiety management – 28 hits ▪ anxiety AND HIV/AIDS – 159 hits ▪ anxiety management AND HIV/AIDS – no hits ▪ anxiety AND immun* – 285 hits ▪ anxiety AND immun* AND HIV/AIDS – 103 hits	The OTseeker search used slightly different search terms to the CINAHL search, because the search facility of OTseeker allows you to identify interventions and diagnosis as well as keywords The search terms used were: ▪ HIV OR AIDS as key words, as neither were identified in the list of diagnoses ▪ relaxation/stress management was the most relevant intervention from the OTseeker list ▪ this combination of key words and a specified intervention produced 14 hits: • 1 of these hits was a systematic review, which was not given a quality score • 13 of the hits were clinical trials, all but one of which had been assigned quality scores

■ Scenario 2.2 ■

Question and search terms

What is the evidence for the value of energy conservation as a means of improving quality of life/occupational performance and decreasing levels of fatigue in clients who experience high levels of fatigue associated with chronic illnesses such as MS, AIDS or RA?

Problem	Intervention	Alternative interventions	Outcome
Fatigue associated with: ■ MS ■ HIV/AIDS ■ RA	Energy conservation	Individual or group session; length of course; handouts and/or discussions; self-help	Improved quality of life; increased occupational performance; decreased fatigue

■ Search terms 2.2 ■

Problem	Intervention	Alternative interventions	Outcome
fatigue multiple sclerosis HIV AIDS rheumatoid arthritis	energy conservation rehabilitation	education groups	activities of daily living quality of life

Choice of databases

This question covers a wide area with both a rehabilitation and medical focus. The databases searched should give access to both medical and allied health literature. The databases chosen for the search were:

■ PubMed
■ AMED

A comparison of these two databases is given in Table 2.3.

Outcomes of search

Of the 537 hits identified by the PubMed searches, only 34 proved to be usefully related to the question, and of those only a small number appeared to be research-based articles. The most useful search was the first, fatigue/rehabilitation search. Many of the items found on this search reappeared on other searches. The lessons to be learnt from this search are to identify the key elements of the question and to use these as the terms for the search, and not to make the search too elaborate by adding new terms just for the sake of including all the possible key terms. If the first terms have been well chosen they should produce the best results.

The results of the AMED search gave 98 hits in total. Of these, 23 were relevant to the question. However, five of these articles appeared in at least two PubMed searches. The two most productive searches were 'fatigue AND rehabilitation' and 'fatigue AND multiple sclerosis'. The success of the various combinations of search terms indicates that, unlike in the PubMed search, the evidence-based occupational therapist should not always be satisfied with the results of the first search terms.

Table 2.3 Search strategy: comparing PubMed and AMED.

PubMed	AMED
Using PubMed's advanced search facility PubMed has a MeSH browser, which allows the searcher to refine the key terms to be used in the search	Following the successful strategy for the PubMed search, 'fatigue' and 'rehabilitation' were chosen as the search terms
From the relatively long list of key terms (Search terms 2.2) an initial search was carried out using the MeSH terms 'fatigue' and 'rehabilitation' and the Boolean operator AND. This search identified 77 hits	When fatigue was reviewed using the thesaurus, it was not an accepted term, alternative terms included: ■ fatigue mental ■ fatigue syndrome chronic ■ muscle fatigue
A further search using 'activities of daily living' AND 'fatigue' gave 46 hits, most of which were duplications of the fatigue/rehabilitation search	Ignoring the thesaurus, fatigue was used as a 'natural word'
Further searches were carried out using the terms: ■ multiple sclerosis ■ rheumatoid arthritis ■ HIV ■ AIDS	Fatigue AND rehabilitation were searched and produced 63 hits
	To ensure that references to the specific illnesses were not being missed, fatigue was combined with: ■ multiple sclerosis – 20 hits ■ rheumatoid arthritis – 9 hits ■ HIV/AIDS – 6 hits
Paired with both 'fatigue' and 'activities of daily living', these searches identified a further 240 references	
PubMed also has the phrase 'see related articles' by each citation; this was accessed for a number of selected articles and produced 174 further hits	

The PubMed search was successful using the MeSH terms. However, the AMED search was more productive when natural language was used. The lesson from this search indicates that there are occasions when the thesaurus should be ignored and natural language should be used as search terms.

■ Scenario 2.3 ■

Question and search terms

What is the evidence for the value of memory aids as a means of decreasing confusion and improving memory function and occupational performance in clients with memory impairment as a result of brain injury?

Problem	Intervention	Alternative interventions	Outcome
Memory impairment following brain injury	Memory aids	Group or individual sessions; education or activity	Decrease in confusion; increase in memory function; increase in occupational performance

■ Search terms 2.3 ■

Problem	Intervention	Alternative interventions	Outcome
brain injury head injury memory	rehabilitation memory aids	education groups	activities of daily living

Choice of databases

Because this question is being used as part of a systematic review, the main evidence should be from RCTs. However, memory dysfunction will also be discussed in social science literature. Databases covering both RCTs and social science literature were chosen for this search:

■ ASSIA
■ Cochrane Library

A comparison of the searches using these databases is given in Table 2.4.

Outcomes of search

The 40 hits in the ASSIA search were all deemed to be useful and appropriate to the question. Because ASSIA includes all types of article (review and research) and all types of research methodology, a wide range of studies was identified, a number of which appeared to be RCTs. There was only one duplication with the Cochrane Library search, indicating the rather limited coverage of OT-specific literature in the Cochrane Library.

The Cochrane Library search identified 70 potentially relevant clinical trials. The results of the first, combined, search identified one highly pertinent RCT. The searcher could have been satisfied with that one piece of information. However, the various paired searches identified a further 10 articles that described RCTs and controlled clinical trials (CCTs) of relevance to the question. The moral of this search is: never be satisfied with the first result – further searches may locate even more useful information.

The two databases used in this search appear to have been well balanced and to have provided a varied selection of references with minimal overlap. This combination of databases indicates the value of using a variety of contrasting databases for any evidence-based search.

■ Scenario 2.4 ■

Question and search terms

What is the evidence for the value of activity as a means of improving mood in clients with depression?

Problem	Intervention	Outcome
Depression	Activity	Improved mood

Table 2.4 Search strategy: comparing ASSIA and Cochrane Library.

ASSIA	Cochrane Library
The key terms used were: ■ memory ■ head injury ■ brain damage/injury 40 hits were identified	The Cochrane Library has both simple and advanced search facilities. This search was carried out using the advanced search facility
	Prior to searching, the MeSH thesaurus was used to refine and identify the most effective search terms
	The following terms were identified as the most relevant terms for this question: ■ head injury ■ memory ■ memory disorders ■ rehabilitation
	When all of the search terms were combined, using the Boolean operator AND, the search produced one hit
	When the various terms were paired, e.g.: ■ head injury AND rehabilitation ■ memory AND rehabilitation a further 69 hits were identified
	All of the hits were located in the Cochrane Controlled Trials Register

■ Search terms 2.4 ■

Problem	Intervention	Outcome
depression	activity; purposeful activity; exercise; rehabilitation	mood

Choice of databases

As the focus of this question is 'purposeful activity', which is a specifically OT concept, databases that were either OT-specific or had included a wide range of OT journals were chosen. The databases used were:

■ OTDBase
■ AMED

Comparison of results obtained using these databases is summarized in Table 2.5.

Outcomes of search

The OTDBase search produced a wide variety of OT-specific references. Of the 31 hits on the 'vocational:leisure' search, three articles could have direct relevance to the question, and three (one of which is in Hebrew) might have relevance to the question. From the miniOTDBase search, of the actual citations given (21), six had direct relevance to the topic. However, if one considers these six references in terms of their acceptability as 'best' evidence, only one article is a report of an experimental study whilst a further three papers report other nonexperimental research findings.

The AMED search resulted in a total of 202 hits. Of these references 14 appeared to be relevant to the topic. Of the apparently relevant articles there were no duplications between the two AMED searches, indicating the value of using a variety of key words and searches within any one database. In terms of the hierarchy of evidence, only three of the identified articles appeared to be RCTs or experimental research and one was a meta-analysis. The remaining citations either gave no methodological information or were for qualitative research, surveys or case studies. Of the 14 identified articles, none were directly related to all aspects of the original evidence-based question. The majority were concerned with exercise or leisure rehabilitation, particularly with patients who had experienced strokes or cardiac problems with related depression.

One of the problems with this search is that one of the key terms, 'activity', is a very vague term, which has a variety of meanings as was shown by the ways the thesaurus broke the term down. The hits tended to focus on leisure activities rather than the more OT notion of therapeutic and purposeful activity, which was the original focus of the question. More details of this search and its results can be found in Taylor (1999).

▨ Scenario 2.5 ▨

Question and search terms

What is the evidence for the value of horticulture as a purposeful activity and means of improving self-esteem and confidence in clients with eating disorders?

Problem	Intervention	Outcome
Eating disorders: ▪ anorexia ▪ bulimia	Horticulture	Improve self-esteem: ▪ increase confidence in self ▪ increase confidence in abilities

▨ Search terms 2.5 ▨

Problem	Intervention	Outcome
eating disorders	horticulture; horticulture therapy gardening; rehabilitation	

Choice of databases

The focus of this question is a therapeutic activity, horticulture. Therefore, the databases to be searched should include a wide range of OT and other therapy references. Horticulture is also a topic of interest beyond healthcare and references and information could be available in a wide range of areas. The databases chosen to search were:

▪ AMED
▪ world wide web

To search the web you need what is known as a 'search engine'. Search engines are internet sites that have an automated search device (known as a 'crawler'). Crawlers search the internet and collect together web pages. The crawler then creates an index and catalogue of all the collected pages. However, the evidence-based occupational therapist should be aware that no attempt is made to review or assess the quality of these web pages. If it is on the web it will be included in the index. When you access a search engine you can search the index by using keywords, just as if

Table 2.5 Search strategy: comparing OTDBase and AMED.

OTDBase	AMED
Because the author, like many occupational therapists, was not a subscriber to OTDBase, access was gained via one of the regular 'open house' months (http://www.otdbase.org)	The key words chosen were: ▪ depression ▪ activity ▪ rehabilitation
The OTDBase preview category 'vocational', which is available to non-subscribers, was chosen	AMED's thesaurus was used to refine the search terms
This category can be linked with other key words – 'leisure' was chosen	New search terms were identified: ▪ depression ▪ depressive disorder ▪ human activity ▪ leisure activities
This search gave 31 hits, each hit included bibliographic information and could be expanded to give the abstract	These were combined using the Boolean operators OR and AND to give a search of depression OR depressive disorder AND human activities OR leisure activities
The miniOTDBase was then searched	
From the table of key words 'activity' was chosen	This search resulted in 98 hits
This gave a series of five subheadings: ▪ analysis ▪ crafts ▪ motivation ▪ research ▪ selection	A second search was carried out using the search terms depression OR depressive disorder AND rehabilitation, to ensure that useful articles had not been missed
For each subheading, the number of possible hits is given plus the full citations and abstracts for the three most recent articles: ▪ research gave 3 potential hits ▪ crafts gave 11 potential hits ▪ motivation gave 38 potential hits	This search resulted in 104 hits
The key word 'mental health' was chosen	
This gave 28 subheadings, of which the most relevant were searched: ▪ activity – 40 hits ▪ depression – 25 hits ▪ programme cost-effectiveness – 3 hits ▪ programme efficacy – 55 hits	

you were searching a database. The search engine will produce a list of *all* the websites in its index that contain the keyword(s). These are known as *hits* and are ranked (by the search engine) according to their relevance to the keyword(s). Relevance is defined by the search engine in terms of factors such as location (i.e. is the word in the title, the abstract, the text) and frequency, which might not translate into relevance for your particular search. However, *be warned*, web searches can produce millions of hits!

There are a number of techniques available for refining web searching, for example:

" " (quotation marks) can be used to make a number of words into a phrase, rather than separate terms, e.g. "occupational therapy" or "horticulture therapy";

+ (plus sign) indicates that a word must be present in all hits, e.g. +horticulture +therapy;

− (minus sign) indicates that a word should be excluded from all hits (e.g. therapy–physical could be used to exclude references to physical therapy/physiotherapy);

* (asterisk) can be used to truncate words where a number of word endings are possible (e.g. therap* would access both therapy and therapist).

Most search engines also have advanced search options where you can use Boolean search operators (e.g. AND, NOT, OR).

A number of search engines and sites exist including:

▪ www.altavista.com
▪ www.yahoo.co.uk
▪ www.excite.co.uk
▪ www.webcrawler.com
▪ www.google.com

AltaVista is commonly regarded as one of the best search engines, because it has a large and comprehensive index, and so was chosen for this search. A further discussion of the use of the internet in evidence-based practice can be found in Chapter 6. A comparison of database searches using AMED and the world wide web is shown in Table 2.6.

Table 2.6 Search strategy: comparing AMED and world wide web.

AMED	World wide web
The search terms used were: ▪ horticulture ▪ horticulture therapy ▪ eating disorders	Using AltaVista's simple search facility
	Using the terms "horticulture therapy" and "eating disorders", the search produced 1 080 000 hits! Note that " " was used to indicate that horticulture therapy and eating disorders should be treated as phrases rather than separate search terms
AMED's thesaurus was used to refine the search terms. This proved interesting as horticulture and horticulture therapy did not exist on the AMED listing; 'gardening' was therefore chosen as an alternative search term, 'eating disorders' was exploded to include all related terms and areas, e.g. anorexia and bulimia	
	As a way of attempting to refine this vast number of hits into something manageable and useful, AltaVista's advanced search facility was used
'Horticulture' was used as a natural language search term and produced 3 hits	The advanced search facility allows the use of Boolean operators and date limits for the search and for the search to be refined by excluding certain search terms
'Gardening' and 'eating disorders' were searched, using the Boolean operator AND, and produced 3 hits	
'Gardening' alone produced 20 hits	Using the advanced search, "horticulture therapy" AND "eating disorders" provided a more modest 37 hits
It was then decided to combine 'eating disorders' and 'rehabilitation' (also exploded) to see if any other relevant articles could be found and this search resulted in 30 hits	Information is displayed on pages containing 10 hits at a time, each item can be expanded to link with the particular website

Outcomes of search

Altogether the AMED search resulted in 56 hits from the various search terms and combinations of eating disorders/gardening/horticulture/rehabilitation. Of the 56 hits, 13 had relevance for the question with only one of these being a duplication (between the horticulture and the gardening searches). None of the identified articles addressed all of the aspects of the original evidence-based question. Articles were either case studies using horticulture in various mental health settings or reviews or case studies of OT with patients with eating disorders. The value of the use of the thesaurus is indicated in this search by the greater number of hits and relevant articles in the 'gardening' search in comparison with the 'horticulture' search – 'gardening' being the word identified in the thesaurus.

Of the 37 sites and web pages identified in the internet search only four had any relevance to the question. The web is a vast resource. However, it tends to be disorganized and idiosyncratic. Although it can allow access to up-to-date information from around the world, it is often a matter of luck that relevant information is accessed. AltaVista is only one of a number of search engines and the researcher may benefit from attempting the same search using a variety of search engines.

The combination of AMED and the web resulted in a number of potential sources of information about horticulture as a therapeutic medium. The lack of research evidence for the value of horticulture therapy and the lack of any references suggesting the use of horticulture with patients with eating disorders indicates that this is a potentially useful area for further research.

■ Scenario 2.6 ■

Question and search terms

> *What information can be derived from a range of evidence into the support needs of people caring for someone who has Alzheimer's disease, in order to facilitate a support group?*

Problem	Intervention	Outcome
Support needs/issues of people caring for someone with Alzheimer's disease	A range of interventions including: ■ support groups ■ group work ■ self-help ■ educational group	Guidelines for facilitating a support group

■ Search terms 2.6 ■

Problem	Intervention	Outcome
Alzheimer's disease; carers	support groups; self-help; educational groups	

Choice of databases

The focus of this search is to find evidence from both qualitative and quantitative research as well as more personal narrative accounts of caring for someone with Alzheimer's disease. The databases searched should give access to a breadth of health and social care research literature as well as other levels of evidence such as experiential accounts. The databases chosen to search were:

Table 2.7 Search strategy: comparing CINAHL and the world wide web.

CINAHL	World wide web
The search terms used were: ▪ Alzheimer's disease ▪ carers ▪ support groups ▪ self-help The various search terms were combined using both AND and OR: ▪ carers AND support groups OR self-help – 173 hits ▪ Alzheimer's disease AND (carers AND support groups OR self-help) – 46 hits	Using Google's advanced search facility, the terms used were: ▪ Alzheimer's disease ▪ carer support groups This search resulted in 162 000 hits!

▪ CINAHL
▪ world wide web

Having used AltaVista for the previous search, it was decided to use another popular search site, namely Google. A comparison of searches using CINAHL and Google is summarized in Table 2.7.

Outcomes of search

By combining the various terms in the CINAHL search, 46 potentially useful papers were identified. By not limiting the search to research papers it was possible to identify opinion pieces and narrative accounts as well as research papers. All of the hits were potentially valuable, and 17 of the hits had direct relevance to the original question. The evidence found included a systematic review, RCTs, qualitative research, opinion pieces and experiential narratives, making this a very useful search.

By contrast the Google search was much less useful. It produced an overwhelming 162 000 hits. The majority proved to be links to the webpages of a variety of support groups, which reinforced the need for support groups but did not yield useful evidence for answering the original evidence-based question.

Whilst the CINAHL search produces a small number of potentially very useful papers, the Google search proved overwhelming, and could reinforce the novice searcher's perception that searching is too difficult as there is too much information available. From the evidence of this search the value of CINAHL as a valuable resource for the evidence-based occupational therapist who wants to access a range of research resources has been soundly reinforced.

Review of the databases

Having given an overview of the various searches, it now seems appropriate to review the various databases used in these searches and to highlight key points to successful searching. All of the databases searched have their strengths and, as indicated above, should be used in combination to provide access to the widest range of evidence. It should be noted that the databases listed below are in alphabetical order and not in order of preference or perceived value. Table 2.8

Table 2.8 Summary of databases.

Database	Coverage	Relevance to occupational therapy*	Rigour of content	Access	Effort required
AMED	Main focus is therapies and rehabilitation	Very relevant	Mixed – must be critically appraised	Should be accessible through healthcare (academic and hospital) libraries	Some training advisable for most efficient use
ASSIA	Focus on social sciences and social aspects of care	Fairly relevant, but highly relevant for some topics	Mixed – must be critically appraised	Should be accessible through academic libraries, may be accessible through health or social care libraries	Some training advisable for most efficient use
CINAHL	Main focus is nursing with some rehabilitation literature	Fairly relevant	Mixed – must be critically appraised	Should be accessible through health care (academic and hospital) libraries	Some training advisable for most efficient use
Cochrane Library	Main focus is RCTs and systematic reviews	Highly relevant for some topics, otherwise of some relevance	High-quality and rigorous information	Should be accessible through healthcare (academic and hospital) libraries	Straightforward, however, some training advisable for most efficient use

OTDBase	OT-specific literature	Highly relevant	Mixed – must be critically appraised	On the internet, by subscription	Straightforward and easy to use
OTseeker	Systematic reviews and clinical trails of relevance to OT	Very relevant	High – all clinical trials are rated for validity and interpretability	OTseeker is available free on the internet	Straightforward and easy to use
PubMed/MEDLINE	Medical focus, although a broad definition of medicine	Fairly relevant	Mixed – must be critically appraised	PubMed is available free on the internet. MEDLINE should be accessible through healthcare (academic and hospital) libraries	Some training advisable for most efficient use
World wide web	Anything and everything!	Limited relevance, but it will depend on the topic	Unknown – needs very careful appraisal	Internet access required	Straightforward, however, some training advisable for most efficient use

*Relevance to OT is defined on a scale as: very relevant; highly relevant; fairly relevant; some relevance; limited relevance.

summarizes the key aspects of each of the databases used in these searches. More detailed information on these databases, together with other sources of evidence, can be found in Chapters 6 and 10.

■ **AMED** – probably one of the best resources for OT intervention and healthcare and social care literature in general. Natural language should be used as search terms in initial searches; only when this is unsuccessful should the thesaurus be used. However, AMED's indexing is not always very thorough and searches may provide fewer hits than expected due to the limitations of the indexing rather than due to lack of published literature. If, for example, you use 'systematic review' as your key words (see Chapter 4 on Systematic reviews) you will access literature reviews as well as *systematic* reviews.

■ **ASSIA** – contains a breadth of social science literature and might be a useful second source of evidence in combination with AMED/Cochrane, etc.

■ **CINAHL** – performed well in comparison with AMED and proved better than the web-based search using Google. CINAHL would be a useful source if the question demanded a greater emphasis on nursing or a broader healthcare literature.

■ **Cochrane Library** – is easy to use and has a good help section, which gives the novice user a clear guide to getting the best out of the Cochrane Library. It is probably the best source for RCTs and CCTs, especially in medicine, but is getting better in its inclusion of OT and OT-related literature.

■ **OTDBase** – this does the key word choosing for you, which might be useful for the novice searcher; however, it does not allow for very specific or sophisticated searches.

■ **OTseeker** – is an excellent resource for the evidence-based occupational therapist who wants to find both systematic reviews and clinical trials that are of direct relevance to OT. Clinical trials are rated in terms of their validity and interpretability. It is possible to search the database using both natural language and predetermined search terms.

■ **PubMed** – is an excellent resource for medical literature, but searches can produce overwhelming numbers of hits. The advanced search facility is very useful. Unlike AMED, PubMed searches should begin with the MeSH thesaurus and only once this is exhausted should natural language be used.

■ **World wide web** – this is a vast resource. However, no attempt has been made to organize information on the web and any search of the web will generate a large number of irrelevant hits and, quite probably, a great deal of frustration.

Pointers for successful searching include:

■ use more than one resource/database;
■ be creative with the key words, and combinations of terms;
■ any search will be limited by the effectiveness of the indexing in any database;
■ any search is only as good as the original question;

- use the thesaurus, but trust natural language first;
- use the advanced search, where possible, to combine terms;
- allow plenty of time;
- search with a 'buddy' (a colleague or friend); two heads will produce more refined search terms and may provide a more critical evaluation of the usefulness of any hit.

Activity

- Refine the question you developed at the end of Chapter 1, identify the key terms and add terms to those you have previously identified.
- Identify your data/information source, which library will you use?
- Work out your budget of time and money available to answer your question.
- Identify possible sources of help with the search, e.g. librarians, students.
- Identify the database(s) that will be most useful for your search.
- Develop your search strategy:
  - refine your search terms;
  - identify the limits to the search:
    — language of article
    — year of publication
    — specific journals
    — research articles only
- Carry out a search.

Accessing evidence

Having completed your search and found a number of useful-looking references, the next task for the evidence-based occupational therapist is to locate the relevant articles. This is not always a simple task. Databases allow access to literature from around the world. However, libraries (even the best-stocked libraries) rarely have access to every journal you might need. Any library, however small, should be able to supply you with most documents. All libraries are part of a network of public, healthcare or academic libraries nationwide.

Nowadays, access to journals is frequently in an electronic format, or e-journals. Libraries will hold paper versions, or hard copies, of some journals but the majority of their holdings of recent and current journals will be accessible electronically, which may require a password, but can mean that searching off-site (from the comfort of your own office or from home) is much easier. If the journal you require is held by the library, it should be possible to print or photocopy the appropriate article. The advantage of this is that you can read the article before you copy it and, therefore, decide if the article really is of relevance to your search. If the library does not have access to the journal you require, it will be able to order a copy of any article either from other libraries in the region. In the UK, copies may be obtained from the British Library, or through the Inter-Library Loan scheme. The thing to remember with any of these methods of accessing articles is that there is a cost involved. Printing and photocopying must be paid for; for example, Inter-Library Loans are usually accompanied by a fee. Therefore, be selective about which references are particularly relevant to your question, otherwise you could be spending a great deal of time and money accessing information that is interesting but not directly relevant to your question.

Possibly the most important resource for any evidence-based occupational therapist is the local librarian. Librarians are experts in dealing with information. They can carry out searches for you or they can help you to carry out your own search. Once the search is completed the librarian can help the evidence-based occupational therapist to access the articles, books and documents required. Most libraries will offer a programme of tutorials and help sessions on:

▪ introduction to the library services;
▪ basic and more advanced searching on a range of databases;
▪ managing references and developing your own database.

Librarians are invaluable sources of knowledge and help. Make friends with your local librarian.

A word about copyright. Copyright is complex and is governed by law. The copyright laws limit the amount of material that can be copied from any published work without the permission of the copyright owner. Infringement of the copyright can lead to prosecution. Copies made by the individual who will be using the material must be for the purposes of research or private study and must not constitute a 'substantial' part of the work. This is interpreted as:

▪ one article from any one issue of a journal;
▪ one chapter from a book.

Activity

▪ Get to know your local librarian, tell them what your areas of interest are and ask them to keep you up to date with information relevant to your areas of interest.
▪ Review the budget you developed above, to include the cost of printing, photocopying and Inter-Library Loans.

Storing and indexing evidence

Having completed the search and acquired all of the relevant material, two tasks remain. The value of the evidence must be appraised (this will be discussed in the following three chapters) and the references and material must be organized and stored. There are three possible options for organizing evidence:

- using folders, files or a filing cabinet to store references, articles and notes;
- using a card index system for references and notes;
- using a personal database to store references and notes.

The only one of these that may be unfamiliar to the reader is probably the personal database approach.

The personal database approach allows you to store references and notes on computer and thus facilitates the creation of reports by allowing material to be copied from the database and incorporated into the report text. Two types of database software are available:

- general databases, such as Access;
- specialist personal bibliographic software (PBS), such as EndNote.

The advantage of PBS software is that it is designed specifically to handle bibliographic information. The disadvantage is the cost of this specialist software. Most personal computers will have some form of preloaded database program included as part of the sales package. General database programs, such as Access, usually have pre-existing templates, which may include a bibliographic database template. This will make creating an evidence-based database somewhat simpler.

Whatever method of organization you choose, you should ensure that the following information is included:

- full bibliographic citation;
- appraisal notes and comments;
- useful quotations, including page reference;
- location of hard copy of article;
- source of original reference.

Activity

- Identify what database software (specialized and general) is available for your use.
- Identify sources of help available to assist your use of the database software.
- Design an organization and storage system.

Further reading and resources

The following further reading and resources will allow the reader to develop a greater knowledge of the various resources available to aid the evidence-based occupational therapist in searching for useful and relevant evidence to underpin practice.

Dale, P. (ed.) (2000) *Guide to Libraries and Information Sources in Medicine and Health Care*, 3rd edn. London: The British Library.

Evidence-Based Occupational Therapy website (http://www.otevidence.info).

Greenhalgh, T. (2006) *How to Read a Paper*, 3rd edn. Oxford: Blackwell Publishing.

Greyson, L. (1997) *Evidence-based Medicine*. London: The British Library.

Reed, K.L. & Cunningham, S. (1997) *Internet Guide for Rehabilitation Professionals*. Philadelphia: Lippincott.

Reynard, K.W. & Reynard, J.M.E. (eds) (2004) *ASLIB Directory of Information Services in the United Kingdom,* 13th edn. London: ASLIB.

ScHARR Introduction to Evidence Based Practice on the Internet (http://www.shef.ac.uk/~scharr/ir/netting.html).

Trawling the Net. A ScHARR Introduction to Free Databases of Interest to NHS Staff on the Internet (http://www.shef.ac.uk/~scharr/ir/trawling.html).

3: Using clinical trials as evidence

It used to be said that randomized controlled trials (RCTs) and controlled clinical trials (CCTs) were not methods used frequently in occupational therapy (OT) research (Taylor 1997). However, this has begun to change. A preparatory search for this chapter revealed 273 RCTs and CCTs listed in the Cochrane Central Register of Controlled Trials when 'occupational therapy' was used as the search term, with the location of the search term limited to inclusion in the abstract of the record. A search of CINAHL using the terms:

'randomized controlled trial' (which the database maps to the term 'clinical trial')

AND

'occupational therapy' (with limits on the search to include only research papers)

revealed 118 hits; a similar search of AMED produced 20 hits. The OTSeeker database listed 3133 RCTs and CCTs at the time of writing this chapter, indicating the growing use of trials to investigate the effectiveness of interventions pertinent to OT, and the growing need for therapists to have the skills critically to appraise the strength of individual trials as evidence. Examples of RCTs relevant to OT will be used to illustrate the various aspects of RCTs throughout this chapter.

Whilst the use of RCTs as a research approach within occupational therapy has increased in recent years, the debate about the value and role of RCT evidence within evidence-based OT has continued, with Clegg and Bannigan (1997), amongst others, arguing strongly for the use of RCTs within evidence-based occupational therapy, and Tse *et al.* (2000) and Hyde (2004) proposing a broader evidence perspective for the effectiveness of OT interventions. This broader perspective of evidence pertaining to OT interventions and actions was discussed in Chapter 1. It is beyond the scope of this introductory text to develop the debate around RCTs in OT, and the further readings identified at the end of this chapter might be a useful starting point for the reader who is interested in exploring this contentious topic further.

RCTs are, however, seen by many in the evidence-based community as the gold standard for evidence of the effectiveness of interventions. Therefore it is important for evidence-based occupational therapists to be able to understand and critically appraise RCTs and CCTs. This chapter will draw on examples of published OT

RCTs to outline the nature of clinical trials. The findings of these trials will then be outlined and used as illustrations to explain the statistical analysis used in RCTs. It is not the intention of this chapter to make the reader a competent data analyst but to enable the reader to read and understand the results section of any research paper, rather than skip over the results and move straight to the discussion. Chaper 10 (Useful resources) includes an annotated bibliography, which will highlight possible sources of further information on research design and analysis.

What are clinical trials?

The aim of any clinical trial is to test the effectiveness of an intervention, whether in comparison with no intervention or with another form of intervention. The most rigorous form of clinical trial is the randomized controlled trial (RCT) (Box 3.1). An alternative, and less rigorous, form of clinical trial is the controlled clinical trial (CCT). Other forms of experimental evidence include the pre-test post-test design and single-subject designs; however, the critical appraisal of these research designs is beyond the scope of this chapter.

> **Box 3.1** Aims and focus of the study
>
> The study of Hammond *et al.* (2004) compared the effect on function, disease, and physical and psychosocial status of a specialized OT intervention with routine care for people with early rheumatoid arthritis (RA). Early RA was defined as RA that had been diagnosed within the past 2½ years. Participants were randomly allocated to the OT or routine interventions groups. Participants receiving the routine interventions did not normally have any intervention from an occupational therapist, physiotherapist or specialist nurse. Participants in the OT intervention group received four 1-hour individual treatment sessions and attended a 2-hour arthritis education group. Participants were assessed, using a variety of specific standardized measures of function and psychosocial status as well as adherence to self-management techniques, at baseline and at 6-months, 12-months and 24-months follow-up.

Randomized controlled trials

Any RCT will consist of a number of phases, as illustrated in Fig. 3.1 and Box 3.4.

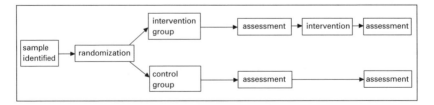

Figure 3.1 Phases of a randomized controlled trial (RCT).

Box 3.2 The process of randomization

The study by Stewart *et al.* (2005) attempted to compare the effectiveness of occupational therapist-led assessments of older people with that of social worker-led assessments. Following referral for assessment, baseline data were collected from both the older person and his or her carer. Data collected included level of dependency and quality of life for the older person and quality-of-life measures from the carer. Participants were then randomly assigned to either the occupational therapist-led assessment group or the social worker-led assessment group. Randomization took place by means of opening the next in a sequence of numbered sealed envelopes. The randomization sequence had originally been generated using random number tables. Participants were then assessed by either an occupational therapist or a social worker. Follow-up data, using the same measures as at baseline, were collected at 4 and 8 months.

The reason RCTs are seen as such useful sources of evidence for assessing the effectiveness of any intervention is because of the process of randomization (Box 3.2). This means that, having decided who the sample population is to be and setting clear parameters for who is acceptable to the trial, each participant has an equal likelihood of being allocated to the intervention group or the control (non-intervention) group. This ensures that any bias is minimized and that the two groups of participants are as similar as possible. Without random allocation of participants, the researcher might choose the 'best' clients to be members of the intervention group. If the participants in the two groups are as similar as possible the research can, then, state with confidence that any differences at the end of the study are due to the intervention and not to differences between the groups. Sometimes, to ensure that the groups are not only similar but properly representative of component variables within the population (e.g. age, level of disability) the sample is 'stratified', or divided into subgroups, before randomization, to allow each subgroup to be fully randomized.

The problem often identified for RCTs as evidence for OT interventions is that by having clear and specific inclusion criteria many trials do not include clients with the breadth and complexity of needs that many occupational therapists come across in everyday practice. It is often difficult, therefore, to see how a particular trial might have relevance for the complexities of OT interventions.

The need for a control group can be seen as ethically problematic, as half of the participants in the trial will be denied a potentially effective intervention. There are a number of approaches to the use of a control group (Box 3.3). The control group may receive: no intervention, as in the Liddle *et al.* (1996) study; the existing intervention, as in the studies of Hammond *et al.* (2004) and Gräsel *et al.* (2005); an alternative intervention, as in the Stewart *et al.* (2005) study; or a combination, as in the Clark *et al.* (1997) study.

The use of an alternative or existing intervention, rather than no intervention, reduces the risks of any placebo effect. The control group provides a baseline against which any changes in the intervention group can be compared to assess whether the intervention has been effective.

Box 3.3 The use of a control group

In a study of the short-term effects of a home environmental intervention on self-efficacy and upset in caregivers and daily function of dementia patients, Gitlin *et al.* (2001) compared the effects of the intervention programme of five home visits from an occupational therapist with the effects of a control group that consisted of educational materials and booklets on environmental safety. Thus, the control group received some of the same information as the intervention group but without the detailed personalized intervention of the occupational therapist.

In a study evaluating OT intervention in maintaining the independence and quality of life of older people, Liddle *et al.* (1996) randomly allocated participants who had been assessed by an occupational therapist as needing equipment/home modifications/services to an intervention or nonintervention group. The intervention group were given the equipment, etc. that had been recommended. The nonintervention group did not have the occupational therapist's recommendations carried out. Clients who were assessed to require no further intervention formed a further control group. Assessment measures included quality of life and functional activity. Participants were reviewed 6 months after the initial interview.

Box 3.4 The phases of an RCT

Whilst many trials consist of three phases (baseline assessment, intervention and follow-up assessment) some trials have more complex designs. The study by Mathiowetz *et al.* (2005) into the effectiveness of an energy conservation course for people with multiple sclerosis (MS) is a case in point. Following initial screening participants were randomly assigned to either the intervention or the control group. Baseline data on function, the impact of fatigue and quality-of-life measures were then collected. The intervention group then received a 6-week energy conservation intervention. Outcome data were then collected. The control group then were given access to the same energy conservation group. Final outcome data were collected from both groups at the end of the 13-week study period.

Controlled clinical trials

Controlled clinical trials (CCTs) also aim to assess the effectiveness of an intervention by comparing two groups of participants (Box 3.5). However, for practical or ethical reasons it is not possible randomly to allocate participants to the respective groups. CCTs often use pre-existing divisions as a way of dividing participants into intervention and control groups, for example, by using participants from different geographical areas or patients on different wards (Gräsel *et al.* 2005).

The phases of a CCT are the same as those of an RCT, in terms of assessment, intervention and reassessment. The problem with any CCT is that the two groups cannot be assumed to be as similar as they would be if randomization had taken place. Any research papers should be appraised carefully to ensure that the groups being compared are similar on all key variables.

Box 3.5 Controlled clinical trials relevant to OT

Gräsel *et al.* (2005) used a CCT to compare the effectiveness of an intensive programme to facilitate the transition from hospital to home for stroke patients and their carers. Following their stroke, patients were admitted to one of two wards. Patients on Ward I experienced the standard approach to the transition from hospital. Patients on Ward II had the standard approach plus additional interventions, such as a psycho-educational seminar for carers, individualized carer training programmes, supported weekend at home before discharge, and access to telephone counselling once the patient had been discharged.

Box 3.6 Inclusion criteria

The study by Mathiowetz *et al.* (2005) on the effectiveness of energy conservation for people with MS had a twofold screening process to ensure that participants met their inclusion criteria. The first part of the screening took place over the telephone and ensured that the participant:

- Had a diagnosis of MS
- Was 18 years of age or older
- Was functionally literate in English
- Experienced fatigue
- Lived independently in the community

Participants who met all of these criteria were then invited for a face-to-face screening interview, which assessed cognitive function to ensure that participants did not have major cognitive deficits.

    People who were excluded from the study were given information on fatigue management.

Ensuring that trials are scientifically rigorous

A number of factors are seen as ensuring that trials are rigorous, that they are measuring what they are supposed to (internal validity), and that the results can be applied to the wider population (external validity). These factors include the use of clear inclusion criteria (Box 3.6) and whether anyone involved in the study (participants, researchers/assessors or therapists) is aware which group the participant is in (blinding).

    RCTs and CCTs are invaluable methods for assessing the effectiveness of a particular intervention with a clearly defined client group or population and applying strict inclusion criteria for who might be included in the study. Both research methods require rigorous standardization of procedures and measures, which will result in objective and statistical analysis of the intervention outcomes. As we have seen, these methods are becoming more frequently used in OT research. However, the more subjective elements are ignored by RCTs and CCTs. RCTs and CCTs will not provide evidence of how the client perceived the intervention or anything about the client's experience of, or satisfaction with, the intervention. RCTs and CCTs will be able to answer the question 'did the intervention work?' These methods of research will not be able to answer the questions 'how was it for the client?' or 'was the client satisfied with the intervention process and outcome?' Only qualitative research methods, which are discussed in Chapter 5, can answer these types of questions.

The magic *P* value: an outline of probability and statistical analysis relevant to appraising RCT evidence

When reading a research paper the part most people dread, and therefore skip over or ignore, is the results section. This section is always full of numbers and symbols, which make little sense to the reader, unless she or he has a sound grasp of statistical concepts. The aim of this part of the chapter is to help you to feel more confident when reading the results section of an RCT report and especially to focus on the key pieces of information needed to appraise an RCT.

Statistical analysis can be divided into two groups. Each group of analysis serves a different function. The first type of analysis is *descriptive analysis*. This allows the researcher to describe the data and to make general observations about the data and the findings. The second type of analysis is *inferential analysis*. This is where the results of the various participant groups are compared, differences between groups are assessed and conclusions are drawn. The main task of inferential analysis is to assess the likelihood of any differences between the groups having occurred by chance. This is referred to as *probability* and is expressed as a *p* value.

Descriptive analysis

One way of describing a participant group is to use *percentages* as a way of indicating what proportions of the group represent different variables or characteristics, for example age, gender, ethnicity, diagnosis, social class.

Another method of describing a population is to use the average, or *mean*. The statistical symbol for the mean is $\bar{x}$. The mean, however, only gives a single figure that describes a middle point in the data. The mean does not give any idea of the overall spread, dispersion and variations of the data. The *range* and the *standard deviation* (SD) give the reader information about the spread and the distribution of scores. The range is the highest and the lowest scores. The standard deviation is a method of describing the spread of scores and how close to the mean the majority (68%) of the scores lie. The larger the standard deviation the greater the spread of scores. Together the mean, range and standard deviation give the reader a clearer overview of the data being presented (Box 3.7).

Box 3.7 The use of descriptive statistics to compare groups of participants

In the study by Hammond *et al.* (2004) of the effectiveness of OT intervention for people in the early stages of RA, the mean age of the OT group was 53.9 years whereas for the control group the mean age was 57.1 years, which might imply that the control group were older than the enhanced group. This was confirmed by statistical analysis, which showed that there was a statistically significant difference between the two group ($p = 0.04$). However, the average duration of the illness was 9 months for both groups. The range of illness duration for the sample was 1–30 months, with almost half of the sample (49%) having had RA for less than 6 months, indicating that many of the participants were in the very early stages of the disease.

In a study by Gitlin *et al.* (2001), of carers of people with dementia, the demographic data were given not only for the participants who completed the study but also for the participants who dropped out of the study before it was completed. This allowed a comparison of all of the participants, and showed that there were no differences between either the intervention/control groups or the participants who completed the study and those who dropped out. The average age of the caregivers was 61, but comparison of the standard deviation (14 years) and the range of ages (23 to 92 years) shows how important it is to have as much information as possible about the measures of variation of the data, otherwise there would be an impression that the majority of the carers within the study were elderly. The amount of time over which the person had been giving care was similarly wide (mean 45 months, SD 34 months, range 2 months to 16 years).

Because the mean can be affected by extreme values, other methods of describing the midpoints or *central tendency* of the data are also used, especially where the data may include extreme values. The most commonly used alternative measure of central tendency is the *median*. This is the actual midpoint if the data were set out in order. Where the data are expressed as a number of categories, for example age bands, social classes or professional groups, then the *mode* is used to describe the category most frequently recorded.

Descriptive analysis can be written in the text of the results, presented in table format (e.g. participant characteristics and demographic information) or displayed in graph or chart form.

Inferential statistics

As mentioned above, the aim of inferential statistics is to compare data from the intervention and the control groups and to determine whether any differences in outcome between these groups would have occurred by chance. In other words, whether the researcher can be certain that the improvement (or change) in the intervention group was due to the intervention or was due to chance factors. How confident the researcher can be in the effectiveness of her/his intervention is referred to as the *level of significance* of the findings. This is expressed in terms of the *p* value. *P* stands for *probability*.

The probability, or likelihood, that any difference between intervention and control groups can be anything between 1.0000 and 0.0000 (see Figure 3.2). The smaller the value of p, the more confident the researcher can be that any differences are not due to chance. Whether the differences are seen and accepted as due to chance is not, however, left to an arbitrary decision by the researcher. Research convention tends to accept 0.05 as the cut-off point. Above 0.05 and results are described as *not significant* (NS), in other words the differences between the groups are regarded as the result of chance. Below 0.05 and the results are described as *significant*, or statistically significant, and the differences are accepted as being not due to chance factors. What a probability value of 0.05 means is that if the study were to be repeated 100 times, in 95 of the studies you would get the same result.

Setting an acceptable level of probability is all about risk, particularly the level of risk the researcher, and the reader, is prepared to accept when considering whether the results of the study are an error. Figure 3.2 illustrates how probability and risk are related.

The researcher should state in the results section what level of significance is being accepted. Liddle *et al.* (1996, p. 576), by saying 'there was no difference at the level of significance 0.01', are indicating that they accept 0.01 (1 in 100) as their cut-off point, as did Hammond *et al.* (2004), whereas Gitlin *et al.* (2001) indicate that 0.05 (1 in 20) is acceptable. Pereira-Maxwell (1998) proposes that to allow interpretation and appraisal of research, the exact p value should be stated rather

---

If a study were repeated, how likely is it that **NO** differences would be found or that any differences between the intervention and control groups would be due to chance factors?

1.0000   0.0000
⊢──⊣
very likely   very unlikely

P value	Likelihood	Ratio
0.80	Very likely	4 in 5
0.50	Pretty likely	1 in 2
0.05	Fairly unlikely	1 in 20
0.01	Pretty unlikely	1 in 100
0.001	Very unlikely	1 in 1000

Figure 3.2 An overview of probability and risk.

than NS (for nonsignificant results) or $p < 0.05$ (for significant results), which is what both Hammond *et al.* (2004) and Stewart *et al.* (2005) did. Stewart *et al.* did not specifically state what level of significance is being accepted, but by careful reading of the results it can be assumed that it is the 0.05 level, as the lowest level of significance is 0.049.

Often the results of a statistical test can be influenced as much by factors within the design of the study as by the outcome of the manipulation of the data. If the outcome measure is insufficiently sensitive in measuring small changes in behaviour, then the differences between the groups will be too small to show a statistically significant difference, even if there appear to be qualitative differences between the participants in the various research groups. This can be compounded by the small sample sizes that are frequently present in OT trials. This can result in what is known as a *type II error*, which is where the study has shown useful differences between the groups but the difference has been shown to be not statistically significant (Ottenbacher & Maas 1999). Thus many trials may appear to provide no evidence to support a particular intervention because of lack of statistical significance, when in fact the intervention may be clinically effective.

The process of determining the P value of any data is through a *statistical test* (Box 3.8). The statistical test will allow a numerical value to be calculated from which the P value can be determined. The types of statistical test are many and various, and include:

- t tests
- χ^2 tests (chi-squared)
- Mann–Whitney U tests
- ANOVA

The type of test used will depend on a number of factors, including the number of participants in each group and the type of data. Any researcher should explain what tests were chosen and the reasoning behind the choice. Further details of statistical analysis can be found in any research or statistics text, such as Armitage

---

Box 3.8 Statistical analysis

Because Stewart *et al.* (2005) had a variety of different types of data; they used a range of statistical tests within their analysis, ranging from χ^2 tests to ANOVA. However, overall they found no significant differences between the occupational therapist-led and the social worker-led assessments. They did find small differences ($p = 0.03$) in favour of the occupational therapist-led assessment for aspects of the quality of life of the carers, and in favour of the social worker-led assessments for carer stress ($p = 0.047$) and amount of caring ($p = 0.049$).

Due to the complexity of both the design and the outcome measures, Mathiowetz *et al.* (2005) used ANOVA in an attempt to tease out which of the many variables might show a difference. Overall, the study found that the impact of fatigue was decreased and aspects of quality of life were increased following participation in an energy conservation group.

et al. (2002). Although the results section of any report will contain a wealth of information, the important aspect for any evidence-based occupational therapist to focus on is the *p* values.

Statistical significance will allow the researcher to accept or reject an intervention or to argue that an intervention might be effective in improving certain outcomes for a particular client group. However, this often gives little indication of the *clinical significance* of the results in terms of the size of the treatment effect.

Statistical significance shows that there is a difference in the outcomes of the interventions between the groups. However, it does not give any indication of how meaningful or useful the outcome might be. For example, a new intervention to improve range of movement and opposition of the thumb may show a significant increase compared with the control group, but if the improvement is still only 5 degrees of movement, this still will not allow for any meaningful use of the thumb or facilitate the ability to hold a pen. Thus there is little *clinical* significance to the intervention.

Statistical significance also does not answer the question 'if I use this intervention, how many patients will I need to treat before I see one improvement?' or 'which patients will benefit most from this intervention?' or 'how much money will this intervention save/cost me?' A result may be statistically significant but be too small to be of value in terms of intervention. Clinical significance and the effectiveness of interventions can be assessed by measures such as confidence intervals, numbers needed to treat, odds ratios and relative risk.

Measures of clinical significance

A *confidence interval* (CI) is a way of estimating where the 'true' result for any population lies. The findings of a study may give results in terms of, for example, a mean improvement score. The confidence interval will allow you to judge the strength of that result in terms of the upper and lower values that are potentially possible for the given result. Confidence intervals are expressed as a percentage, with 95% being the most commonly used. The narrower the distance, or interval, between the values the more confident you can be in the result (Box 3.9).

Box 3.9 Using confidence intervals

Liddle *et al.* (1996) compared the percentage of people in the intervention group and the control group who had maintained satisfactory levels of outcomes. The confidence intervals for each figure were also recorded. Thus in the intervention group, 64% of participants maintained a satisfactory score on the Life Satisfaction Index. The 95% confidence interval for this figure was 50 to 78. In other words, the 'true' result could be anything from 50% to 78% of participants maintaining a satisfactory Life Satisfaction Index score.

Findings can also be expressed in terms of *relative risk*. This is a measure of assessing the 'risk' or likelihood of a given event for one group of participants compared with another group (Pereira-Maxwell 1998). If there is no difference in risk between the groups the relative risk value is 1. If the risk is lower for the intervention group the value is less than 1 and greater than 1 if the risk is higher.

Numbers needed to treat (NNT) is a way of measuring the impact of an intervention in terms of how many people need to be treated in order to prevent one negative outcome (Pereira-Maxwell 1998). In other words, an NNT of 25 would mean that for every 25 patients treated one patient would be spared from the negative or adverse effect. Sackett *et al.* (1997) cite the example of intensive insulin therapy as a means of preventing neuropathy in diabetic patients. The evidence suggests an NNT of 15, which would mean that for every 15 diabetic patients treated with an intensive insulin regime one patient would be spared from developing diabetic neuropathy. Thus, the smaller the NNT the more effective the intervention.

A final measure of clinical significance is the *odds ratio* (OR). This measure is more commonly seen in systematic reviews and meta-analyses. Chapter 4 discusses systematic reviews and will include an explanation of odds ratios.

Before we consider how to appraise an RCT as a source of evidence, it is worth noting the effect that publication bias might have on the availability of RCT evidence (Gray 2001). Some journals will only publish research where the results have achieved a 0.05 level of statistical significance. This means that research where the findings are not significant will not be published. This could mean that valuable evidence of the ineffectiveness of interventions is not published.

Appraising clinical trials

The focus of this chapter, and the following chapters on systematic reviews and qualitative research, is to provide the evidence-based occupational therapist with the skills needed critically to appraise research evidence. However, this focus on critical appraisal begs two questions:

- What is critical appraisal?
- Why is critical appraisal of research evidence necessary?

Critical appraisal allows the evidence-based occupational therapist the opportunity to assess the value and trustworthiness of a piece of research within the context of practice and within a structured framework. The structure of the critical appraisal process allows the evidence-based OT to review not just the findings of the research but the whole research process. It is, however, important to bear in mind that no research or research paper is without its flaws. Critical appraisal does not mean taking a research paper apart and spitting out the bits! The flaws of the research should be weighed and evaluated carefully but should be viewed in the context of whether the flaws make you question the conclusions of the researchers. Critical appraisal should be positive rather than negative. Research should be read with an open mind and the ability to challenge your own, as well as the researcher's, ideas and assumptions.

Using a critical appraisal approach to reading research literature will encourage the evidence-based occupational therapist not to ignore, or skip over, the 'complicated' (results) sections of a research paper. Skipping over parts of an article may lead to misinterpretation of findings or accepting (or rejecting) the author's conclusions based on an inaccurate, or incorrect, interpretation of the research. Critical appraisal is often more interesting if it is not a solitary activity, so that the findings and ideas can be discussed and ideas and comments can be challenged and reviewed. Chapter 7 will discuss how journal clubs can be used as a way of sharing critical appraisals of research literature.

The appraisal of any article should address three broad areas:

■ Are the results valid?
■ What are the results?
■ How will these results help me work with my clients?

The first area asks questions that will help you to appraise the rigour of the research and to ask the question 'is this good research?' The second area will ask questions that help you to assess the significance, both statistical and clinical, of the results. The final area enables you to reflect on whether the findings of the research have any direct relation or impact on your areas of OT practice.

Table 3.1 gives an overview of the questions to ask when appraising an RCT. These questions are based on a number of sources, including the questions developed as part of the Critical Appraisal Skills Programme (CASP) initiative and the CONSORT statement (Moher et al. 2001) with some additions, which the author felt were relevant to evidence-based OT[1] (see Chapter 10 for more information about the CASP programme). The CONSORT statement was developed as a way of improving the quality of published reports of RCTs to ensure that published research was clear and transparent and that readers of the research were able to assess the strengths and limitations of any RCT. The CONSORT statement consists of a checklist of 22 items and a flow diagram for reporting an RCT.

The use of a checklist, or series of questions, as a useful tool for critically appraising literature has been advocated by a number of authors, including Strauss et al. (2005), Gray (2001) and Greenhalgh (2006). The various questions will now be expanded, and Table 3.2 gives a worked example of a critical appraisal of an RCT (Ward et al. 2004).

Are the results valid?

Did the trial address a clearly focused issue?

Was there a clearly stated aim to the research? Is the research attempting to address a clear research question? Does the research paper give a clear explanation

---

[1] Other examples of appraisal checklists for RCTs can be found at CASP (http://www.phru.org.uk/~casp/resources/SRfrontpage.htm).

Table 3.1 Questions to ask when critically appraising a clinical trial.

Are the results valid?
■ Did the trial address a clearly focused issue?
■ Was the assignment of participants to treatments randomized?
■ Were all the participants who entered the trial properly accounted for at its conclusion?
■ Is the literature review appropriate?
■ Were participants, health workers and study personnel 'blind' to the treatment?
■ Were the groups similar at the start of the trial?
■ Apart from the experimental intervention, were the groups treated equally?
■ Were ethical issues considered?

What are the results?
■ Was there an adequate description of the data collection methods used?
■ Were the methods of analysis appropriate, clearly described and justified?
■ What are the key findings?
■ How significant were the results?
■ Have the research aims/question/hypotheses been addressed?

How will the results help me work with my clients?
■ Can the results be applied to the local population of my practice and clients?
■ Were all the important outcomes considered?
■ Are the benefits of the intervention worth any harms and costs?

of the population being studied (this should include the criteria used for inclusion and exclusion of participants to the study)? Does the paper give a clear overview of what interventions were being compared? Does the paper give a clear overview of the outcomes being measured and why those outcomes, and specific outcome measures, were chosen? At the end of reading the paper you should have a clear picture of who was being studied, what was being done to them and what the context of the study was.

Was the assignment of participants to treatments randomized?

The aim of this appraisal is to review RCTs. Therefore, a key question is whether participants were randomly assigned to the various groups. The paper should give a clear explanation of how the randomization took place. If not, the paper is not an RCT and cannot be seen as 'gold standard' evidence.

Were all the participants who entered the trial properly accounted for at its conclusion?

Whilst x number of participants may begin the study it is usually the case that y number of participants complete the study, especially if there is a prolonged follow-up phase. Participants move on, change circumstances or die. However, it is important that all participants are accounted for in some way as part of the analysis. If the researchers fail to do this, the results may be biased.

Table 3.2 Worked example of a critical appraisal of an RCT: Ward, C.D., Turpin, G., Dewey, M.E. *et al.* (2004) Education for people with progressive neurological conditions can have negative effects: evidence from a randomized controlled trial. *Clinical Rehabilitation* **18**, 717–725.

Question	Yes, no, can't tell	Comments
Are the results valid?		
Did the trial address a clearly focused issue?	Yes	The research had a clear objective:
		To test the effects of a home-based education intervention in reducing the incidence and the risks of falls and pressure sores in adults with progressive neurological conditions.
		However, it could be argued that looking at two such different outcomes as falls and pressure sores might mean that the scope of the study is very broad. The fact that the study appears to have found negative rather than positive effects for the intervention might, however, be seen as sufficient grounds to continue with the appraisal and discussions. The population is clearly stated:
		Patients who had progressive neurological conditions were recruited via GPs. The majority of the participants had either MS or Parkinson's disease (PD).
		Outcomes and outcome measures were clearly defined:
		The focus was on self-report of falls and pressure sores. Additional outcome information was collected using standardized measures such as the Nottingham Extended Activities of Daily Living scale (NEADL) and the General Health Questionnaire.
		It was assumed that the reader was familiar with these measures, so no detail was given about the measures.
Was the assignment of participants to treatments randomized?	Yes	Potential participants were identified by their GPs and identified as eligible for the study. These potential participants were then contacted and asked if they were willing to take part in the trial. Participants who agreed were then asked to give written consent to be involved in the study. Following a baseline assessment, participants were then randomly allocated to the two study groups (educational group or comparison group). Randomization was by the use of computer-generated random numbers and the sample was stratified into five diagnostic groups.

Table 3.2 *Continued.*

Question	Yes, no, can't tell	Comments
Were all the participants who entered the trial properly accounted for at its conclusion?	Yes	A clear flow-chart of the participants through the study is given. People consenting to participate in the study totalled 114 and were evenly divided into the two groups (57 in each group). In the educational group 53 participants completed the trial (one person died and three were lost to follow-up) and in the comparison group 52 completed (three people died and two were lost to follow-up).
If the answers to these three screening questions are 'yes', it is worth carrying on with the appraisal		
Is the literature review appropriate?	Yes	Although the Introduction is brief, it does provide an adequate background to the study and its context.
Were participants, health workers and study personnel 'blind' to the treatment?	Can't tell	It is not stated whether the participants were aware which group they had been allocated to. The research occupational therapist carried out the intervention in the educational group and also visited the control group to deliver the information pack, so was not blind to the groupings. It is unclear who carried out the follow-up data collection and so blinding is uncertain. This highlights the complexity of blinding. within therapy intervention trials.
Were the groups similar at the start of the trial?	Yes	A table in the text outlines the comparisons between the two participant groups. They were compared by: ▪ Age ▪ Diagnosis ▪ Sex ▪ Ethnicity ▪ Educational level ▪ Social class ▪ Percent living alone ▪ Years since diagnosis ▪ Falls in previous 12 months ▪ Skin sores in previous 12 months.

(Continued)

Table 3.2 *Continued.*

Question	Yes, no, can't tell	Comments
		Statistical comparisons between the groups were not calculated, but for the majority of baseline characteristics there did not appear to be major differences. However, the education group had experienced more falls in the previous 12 months (31 compared with 22; not a significant difference, $p = 0.144$) and the comparison group had more skin sores over that period (six in comparison to three). No baseline data of ADL function were given in the baseline comparison table (it did appear in a later table). Therefore, it was difficult to assess whether the groups were functionally similar at the start of the study.

Apart from the experimental intervention, were the groups treated equally?	Yes	The baseline information for each member of the educational group was presented to an expert panel, consisting of a range of healthcare professionals. The panel suggested interventions for each participant. Each participant in the educational group then received a visit from the research occupational therapist, who provided:
		■ Personalized advice and information
		■ An information package
		■ A leaflet on self-help organizations specific to the participant's diagnosis
		■ An action plan
		■ A follow-up phone call 2 weeks later to reinforce the educational content of the visit.
		  The comparison group was visited by the research occupational therapist, who delivered an information pack. Any concerns raised by participants were referred back to the GP.
		  No other information was given about what else might be happening to the participants throughout the trial.
		  This highlights not only the complexity of OT interventions but also the complexity of carrying out controlled studies in real-world settings.

Table 3.2 *Continued.*

Question	Yes, no, can't tell	Comments
Were ethical issues considered?	Can't tell	The issue of consent was discussed. However, other ethical issues, such as confidentiality, distress, etc. were not discussed. The control group was not being denied intervention and members were told to contact their GP for further help and advice.
What are the results?		
Was there an adequate description of the data collection methods used?	Yes	The outcome measures used (see above) were standardized, commonly used assessments. A clear overview of the data collection process was given.
Were the methods of analysis appropriate, clearly described and justified?	Yes	The analysis is appropriate and some attempt has been made to outline why particular methods of analysis were chosen.
What are the key findings?		A table provides a clear overview of the comparison in the numbers of falls and skin sores the two groups at 12-month follow-up, with the educational group experiencing more falls and more skin sores. Analysis of the other outcome measures showed that the educational group became less independent, as indicated by the rise in their mean NEADL scores, with PD participants being the subgroup who were responsible for this increase in scores.
How significant were the results?		The difference in reported falls was significant ($p = 0.036$); the difference in reported skin sores was also significant ($p = 0.039$). However, neither of these are highly significant differences, representing a 3 in 100 likelihood of the results occurring by chance. The increases in NEADL scores are much more significant at $p = 0.001$ for the changes in the educational group and participants, 0.003 for the PD subgroup of participants, indicating that the decreases in functional ability experienced by these participants is unlikely to have occurred by chance.

(Continued)

Table 3.2 *Continued.*

Question	Yes, no, can't tell	Comments
Have the research aims/ question/hypotheses been addressed?	Yes	The aim of the study was to explore the impact of an educational programme on the occurrence of falls and pressure sores in people who have progressive neurological conditions. The study found, somewhat surprisingly, that the educational programme appeared to have a negative effect, in that participants in the educational group reported more falls than those in the comparison group at the follow-up stage. However, these findings must be viewed with a degree of caution as the participants in the educational group also appear to have become less independent throughout the course of the study, with this decrease of function having the greatest impact on participants with PD, who might be considered the group most likely to fall.
How will the results help me work with my clients?		*The answers to these questions can only, really, be given by you, the reader, in relation to your service.* *These are my reflections only.*
Can the results be applied to the local population of my practice and clients?		In the light of the recent National Service Framework for Long-term Conditions and the emphasis on falls prevention, this study provides interesting food for thought for any occupational therapist planning both falls prevention and educational programmes for clients with progressive neurological conditions.
		The range of participants in the study is probably representative of the types of clients that might be seen by an occupational therapist working in this area.
Were all the important outcomes considered?		The focus of the trial was on falls and skin sores and these were measured by self-report, which may not be the most accurate way of recording this information. The use of the NEADL provided useful data about the participants' functional abilities, and is a standardized measure. The inclusion of the General Health Questionnaire does not appear to have added any meaningful information to the finding.

Table 3.2 *Continued.*

Question	Yes, no, can't tell	Comments
Are the benefits of the intervention worth any harms and costs?		This is a cautionary piece of research, as it demonstrates that an intervention that many see as beneficial, namely patient education, may not be beneficial and may actually cause harm. This is a useful message to learn for the evidence-based practitioner.
		This study calls into question the efficacy and wisdom of educational and self-management interventions (such as the Expert Patient Programme). As an evidence-based practitioner I would need to explore the topic further before I could say that I had sound evidence of the effects (beneficial or otherwise) of educational programmes for clients with progressive neurological conditions (particularly PD).

It is becoming common for researchers to include a flow diagram, indicating the process of the trial and how many participants were included for each phase of the process. Figure 3.3 shows an example of a flow diagram from a published research study.

The questions above should be used as a screening process to assess the overall value of the research. If the answers to these questions are negative the rigour of the research is questionable and there will be little value in continuing to appraise the piece of research.

Is the literature review appropriate?

Does the literature provide a clear, comprehensive and up-to-date background to the research? Has literature been drawn from a wide range of sources? If the literature review is narrow and reliant on limited sources it may also reflect an underlying preconception and bias on the part of the researcher.

Were participants, health workers and study personnel 'blind' to the treatment?

Being 'blind' means being unaware of the nature of the research. One way of reducing potential bias or confounding influences is to ensure that the people involved in the research are blind. It would be unethical for participants to be unaware that they were part of a research programme. However, it is possible for participants to be unaware of whether they are in the intervention or the control group. It is a well-accepted fact that if participants know they are part of a study

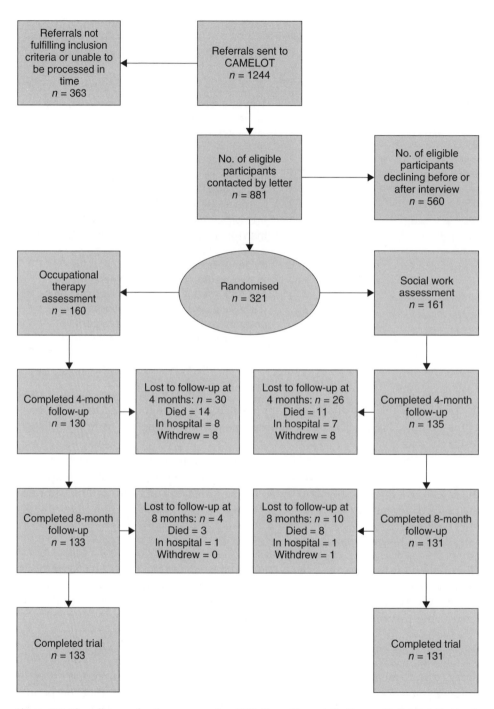

Figure 3.3 Flow diagram for the process of an RCT. (From Stewart, S., Harvey, I., Poland, F., Lloyd-Smith, W., Mugford, M. & Flood, C. (2005) Are occupational therapists more effective than social workers when assessing frail older people? Results of CAMELOT, a randomised controlled trial. *Age and Ageing* **34**(1), 41–46. Reproduced with permission from Oxford University Press.)

this might influence their behaviour. This is known as the Hawthorne effect (Bailey 1997; DePoy & Gitlin 2005). The researchers, especially those carrying out any assessment or outcome measurement, should also be blind as the research process can influence them. The effect on the assessors is called the Rosenthal effect. However, the reader should also note that it may be difficult or unethical in some circumstances for those involved in the research to be blind to the nature of the research.

Were the groups similar at the start of the trial?

The premise of randomization is that all variables are equally distributed between the groups. The groups should, therefore, be similar in terms of relevant factors such as age, gender, social class, ethnicity and length of stay in hospital, as well as for the study's baseline measures. Statistical analysis should be used to establish that there are no significant differences between the groups, and detailed demographic and baseline profiles of the groups should be presented as part of the results.

If there do appear to be differences in the baseline measures for the groups it is your job as the reader/appraiser to decide whether these differences are likely to impact on the outcomes of the research. For example, does it matter that the experimental group had a lower average Barthel Activities of Daily Living (ADL) score than the control group?

Apart from the experimental intervention, were the groups treated equally?

This question relates to two aspects of the research. Firstly, how many people were involved in giving the intervention to the intervention group. If more than one person was involved, was the process of intervention clearly standardized between the different personnel. The second aspect relates to how the control group was treated. If the control group was receiving the 'usual' or 'normal' intervention, was this standardized. Differences in intervention within the various study groups may act as a confounding factor to influence the results.

Were ethical issues considered?

Ethical issues include informed consent, confidentiality, risk factors, denial of or withholding of treatment, or distress caused to the participants. The researchers should discuss how these issues have been dealt with within the study.

What are the results?

Was there an adequate description of the data collection methods used?

The process of data collection should be clearly described. Were the measures used in the study valid and reliable tools for assessing the relevant outcomes? Were the measures sufficiently sensitive to record changes as a result of the intervention? If the measures are not sensitive, then the fact that there is no difference at the end of the study might say more about the outcome measure than about the potential effectiveness of the intervention. All outcome measures should be referenced and a review of their validity and reliability should be given. If new measures have been developed and used in the study, have these been subjected to a rigorous assessment of their reliability and validity?

Were the methods of analysis appropriate, clearly described and justified?

Did the analysis relate to the aims and research questions? Was the choice of statistical analysis explained with a clear rationale for the choice of tests?

What are the key findings?

Do these results answer the research questions? Each outcome measure should be analysed and the results presented, with clear comparisons between the groups.

How significant were the results?

If there are significant differences between the groups, how large are the differences? If confidence intervals are given, how narrow are they? Can the differences be assessed in terms of their clinical significance and value in terms of meaningful improvement?

Have the research aims/question/hypotheses been addressed?

Go back to the aims, research question and hypotheses, which should have been stated at the beginning of the paper. Has the research clearly addressed all these aspects? Has the analysis adequately attempted to interpret the findings in terms of both the research question and the research hypotheses? Have the hypotheses been adequately tested?

How will the results help me work with my clients?

Can the results be applied to the local population of my practice and clients?

Consider the nature of the study's participants; how similar are they to your client group? If the study is of inpatients, how well can this be applied to an outpatient or community setting? Do you have the skills necessary to use the intervention or do you need further skills and training? Would it be possible or appropriate to apply the findings of the study to your work setting?

Were all the important outcomes considered?

Any research can only measure a limited number of outcomes. However, has the research measured the outcomes you feel are the most relevant? If other outcomes should have been considered, do you need to find more evidence before changing your current intervention?

Are the benefits of the intervention worth any harms and costs?

The paper may not address this question. However, you will need to consider the implications of changing your practice, not only for yourself but also for your clients and your purchasers.

▪ ▪

Activity

▪ Identify an RCT relevant to your area of practice/interest.
▪ Using the appraisal questions above, work with a colleague to appraise the article and to assess its value as evidence.

▪ ▪

Further reading

The following references will allow the reader to explore the nature and scope of experimental research in more depth, and to explore the debate about the value of RCT evidence within evidence-based occupational therapy.

Armitage, P., Berry, G. & Matthews, J.N.S. (2002) *Statistical Methods in Medical Research*, 4th edn. Oxford: Blackwell Science.

Bailey, D.M. (1997) *Research for the Health Professional*, 2nd edn. Philadelphia: FA Davis Co.

Clark, F., Azen, A.P., Zemke, R., Jackson, J., Carlson, M., Mandel, D., Hay, J., Josephson, K., Cherry, B., Hessel, C., Palmer, J. & Lipson, L. (1997) Occupational therapy for independent living older adults. *Journal of the American Medical Association* **278**(16), 1321–1326.

Clegg, A. & Bannigan, K. (1997) Shifting the balance of opinion: RCTs in occupational therapy. *British Journal of Occupational Therapy* **60**, 510–512.

DePoy, E. & Gitlin, L.N. (2005) *Introduction to Research*, 3rd edn. St Louis: Mosby.

Greenhalgh, T. (2006) *How to Read a Paper*, 3rd edn. London: BMJ Publishing Group.

Hyde, P. (2004) Fool's gold: examining the use of gold standards in the production of research evidence. *British Journal of Occupational Therapy* **67**(2), 89–94.

Jadad, A. (1998) *Randomised Controlled Trials*. London: BMJ Books.

Moher, D., Schutz, K.F. & Altman, D.G. (2001) The CONSORT statement: revised recommendations for improving the quality of reports of parallel-group randomised trials. *Journal of the American Medical Association* **285**, 1987–1991.

Pereira-Maxwell, F. (1998) *A–Z of Medical Statistics*. London: Arnold.

Robson, C. (2002) *Real World Research*, 2nd edn. Oxford: Blackwell.

Tse, S., Blackwood, K. & Marrolee, P. (2000) From rhetoric to reality: use of randomised controlled trials in evidence-based occupational therapy. *Australian Occupational Therapy Journal* **47**(4), 181–185.

4: Systematic reviews

Systematic reviews, as we discussed in Chapter 1, have been identified as occupying the highest level within the traditional medical hierarchy of evidence. This chapter will explore the nature and value of systematic reviews of research evidence and will discuss the various factors that ensure any systematic review provides high-quality evidence for the evidence-based occupational therapist. The ways of presenting data and findings in systematic reviews and meta-analyses will be outlined, with relevant examples as illustrations. The chapter will conclude by outlining how systematic reviews can be appraised and used to answer evidence-based questions.

Systematic reviews aim to summarize all the available and relevant research on a particular topic; they should also explore and evaluate the quality of any research that is included in the review. The need for systematic reviews has developed because of the vast increase in the volume of health and social care literature over the last two decades. It is impossible for the evidence-based occupational therapist to keep up with all of this material. Equally, there may be a number of studies on the same topic that appear to contradict each other or to produce inconclusive findings. Systematic reviews are a way of exploring the findings and merits of a number of studies and producing a summary of current best evidence on a particular topic.

Whilst randomized controlled trials (RCTs) are seen by many as the 'gold standard' for evidence of the effectiveness of interventions, as we have seen in Chapter 3, the results of an RCT may not be significant or may be statistically significant without being *clinically* significant. The problem with many RCTs is that they are based on small numbers of participants and the likelihood, therefore, of a highly significant result is reduced. However, if the findings from a number of RCTs can be combined and reanalysed, the results may be far more clinically significant and the evidence of the effectiveness of the intervention becomes much stronger. This is the purpose and value of systematic reviews and meta-analyses. In the traditional medical hierarchy of evidence (see Chapter 1), systematic reviews and meta-analysis of RCTs are at the top of the hierarchy and form the highest level of evidence.

Systematic reviews and meta-analyses of occupational therapy (OT) interventions are still relatively rare, although the number of reviews of relevance to OT is growing. A search of CINAHL using the search:

'systematic review AND occupational therapy'

with both terms mapped onto the MeSH terms in the thesaurus, produced just 10 hits, of which only one (Steultjens *et al.* 2005) was a published systematic review. Whilst a similar search using:

'meta-analysis AND occupational therapy'

as mapped terms, produced only one hit for an abstract from the College of Occupational Therapists 2003 Annual Conference. CINAHL was then searched again using:

'systematic review' AND 'occupational therapy'

as natural language. This search resulted in 49 hits, the majority of which were relevant published systematic reviews. A similar repeat search using:

'meta analysis' AND 'occupational therapy'

as natural language resulted in 25 hits, the majority of which had already been identified in the previous natural language search.

A search of the Cochrane Library had mixed results. A search using the MeSH term 'occupational therapy' revealed five hits on the Cochrane Database of Systematic Reviews and 21 hits on the Database of Abstracts of Reviews of Effectiveness (DARE) Abstracts of Quality Assessed Systematic Reviews listing; the location of 'occupational therapy' as a search term was limited to its appearing in either the title, the abstract or the key words. The DARE reviews give a succinct overview and appraisal of the aims, process and findings of any review, as well as an evaluation of the quality of the review. A 'simple' search of the Cochrane Library using 'occupational therapy' produced the same 21 hits on DARE and 12 hits on the Cochrane Database of Systematic Reviews. The Cochrane Database hits included nine completed reviews and three protocols. The completed reviews included:

- occupational therapy for Parkinson's disease;
- occupational therapy for rheumatoid arthritis;
- occupational therapy for multiple sclerosis;
- cognitive rehabilitation for people with schizophrenia and related conditions.

Protocols for reviews of interest currently being conducted included:

- occupational therapy and physiotherapy for developmental coordination disorder;
- occupational therapy for patients with problems in activities of daily living after stroke;
- rehabilitation for distal radial fractures in adults.

Whilst the findings of these searches would appear to support my conjecture that systematic reviews are relatively uncommon in OT, a search of OTSeeker showed that 931 systematic reviews are listed on that database and are, therefore, seen as having relevance to OT.

As well as demonstrating the somewhat limited number of systematic reviews covering occupational therapy interventions specifically, these searches have also added to the lessons learnt in Chapter 2. The CINAHL search demonstrated the value of using Boolean operators, such as AND, to expand search terms. Both the CINAHL and the Cochrane searches demonstrated the limitations of relying solely on MeSH terms at the expense of natural language. Montori *et al.* (2005) have provided a thorough and useful overview of search strategies for locating systematic reviews within the medical context.

Whilst systematic reviews and meta-analyses are relatively rare within OT at the moment, in spite of Ottenbacher's (1983) support for systematic reviews and meta-analysis in OT, they are seen by many as the sources of the highest-level evidence for the effectiveness of interventions.

The systematic reviews used as illustrations within this chapter come from a range of sources and cover a variety of research methodologies. Steultjens *et al.* (2004) is a Cochrane review of the effectiveness of OT interventions for people with rheumatoid arthritis; Barras (2005) is a review of the effectiveness of OT home assessments and draws on a wide range of types of research evidence; and Steultjens *et al.* (2005) is a systematic review of reviews of OT interventions for a variety of different conditions.

Overview of systematic reviews

All researchers know the value of reviewing the existing literature on a given topic. These surveys of existing literature often lead to narrative reviews of the literature. This is where the research findings for a given topic are presented in some form of overview format. The various studies and their findings are often presented in table format. However, little attempt is made to reanalyse the findings within a narrative review. This may be because a variety of research techniques have been employed and direct comparisons cannot be made. A further limitation of the narrative review is that there is often subjectivity involved in the selection of the articles for inclusion or exclusion from the review (Cusick 1986). Whilst narrative reviews can provide interesting food for thought, they rarely provide high-quality evidence.

Systematic reviews aim to improve upon narrative by using rigorous methods to find and review research evidence. Langhorne and Dennis (1998) propose three roles for systematic reviews:

▪ to provide the most reliable summary of available information and research on a given intervention;
▪ to provide invaluable pointers for future research;
▪ reviews may also provide the best estimate of whether a particular intervention is effective.

The aim of any systematic review is to synthesize the findings of all the available appropriate evidence and to do so scientifically, rigorously and without bias.

Box 4.1 The scope of the review

Both Steultjens *et al.* (2004) and Steultjens *et al.* (2005) are broad reviews. The stated objective of Steultjens *et al.* (2004, p. 2) was 'to determine whether occupational therapy interventions for rheumatoid arthritis patients improve outcome on functional ability, social participation and/or health-related quality of life' and so is attempting to review evidence for the breadth of OT interventions for people with rheumatoid arthritis, rather than focus on one aspect, such as splinting or joint protection.

The scope of Steultjens *et al.* (2005) is even broader because it is to summarize the research available from systematic reviews of the efficacy of OT in general terms and for the benefit of a variety of stakeholders including for practitioners, researchers, purchasing organizations and policy-makers. Thus it highlights the value of systematic reviews for guiding not only professional practice but also policy development.

The review of Barras (2005, p. 326) had a much narrower focus on one particular intervention utilized by occupational therapists. Her aim was to 'identify, collate and assess the findings of the available literature regarding discharge planning involving occupational therapy home assessments and the identified outcomes' and to clarify the benefit of the OT home assessment as well as identifying the future research directions for this particular area of practice.

As with all research, systematic reviews follow a clear process (de Vet *et al.* 1997; Langhorne & Dennis 1998; Petticrew & Roberts 2006). Whilst the majority of systematic reviews are solely reviews of experimental and trials-based research (most commonly RCTs) in order to address questions about the effectiveness of interventions, there is a growing discussion of the value of including qualitative research into reviews (Petticrew 2001; Thomas *et al.* 2004; Petticrew & Roberts 2006) and of having reviews that focus solely on qualitative research (e.g. Kylma 2005; Shaw *et al.* 2005).

The systematic review should begin with a clear objective and research question (Box 4.1). This will guide and frame the review. If the question is too broad the reviewers may be overwhelmed with research that is difficult to synthesize and interpret. If the topic is too narrow this may result in limited numbers of relevant research papers being identified and an inability to draw clear conclusions.

Having defined the question, the reviewers must then carry out a comprehensive search of all potentially relevant sources of information. This should ensure that all relevant research studies are located and can be included in the review. Searches should include both computer and hand searches. Relevant databases and internet sites should be identified for computer searches. A comprehensive search strategy, including the identification of key terms, should be developed for the computer searches (Box 4.2). Relevant journals, conference proceedings and current awareness literature should be identified for hand searching. Other relevant sources of information, such as specialist libraries and specialists and experts in the relevant fields, should also be identified.

Box 4.2 The search strategy

Barras (2005) identified her search terms as:

- occupational therapy
- discharge OR discharge planning
- home environment OR home assessment OR home visit
- outcome measure
- elderly OR age OR geriatric OR older

which were use with a number of databases including:

- AMED
- Austhealth
- CINAHL
- Cochrane
- MEDLINE

She also used citation tracking (i.e. following up references cited in selected articles). Hand searching of these collections and conference abstracts was also carried out. Thirty-one papers were identified for possible inclusion in the review.

Steultjens *et al.* (2004) used methods devised by the Cochrane Collaboration Musculoskeletal Group to guide their search. Their search terms for occupational therapy interventions included:

- ADL
- self-help devices
- splints
- patient education
- counselling
- exercise therapy
- self-care
- assistive technology

These terms were used on a range of databases including:

- MEDLINE
- CINAHL
- Embase
- Cochrane Controlled Trials Register

Reference lists were scanned and authors of selected papers were contacted to identify any unpublished studies. The search produced a list of 2694 citations.

Steultjens *et al.* (2005) used the terms 'occupational therapy' and 'review' to search PubMed and the term 'occupational therapy' to search the Cochrane Database of Systematic Reviews and the Database of Abstracts of Reviews of Effectiveness. These searches identified a total of 581 potential references.

A review protocol should be developed. This will outline the criteria to be used for deciding whether studies will be included or excluded from the review (Box 4.3). The criteria should include the types of participants, types of interventions, outcome measures, types of studies and methodological quality criteria. The

Box 4.3 Inclusion criteria

The inclusion criteria of Barras (2005) were quite general and related to whether the papers reported on OT and home assessments and related to patients in acute or rehabilitation hospital settings. The only exclusion criteria were research related to paediatric or mental health settings. No studies were excluded based on the type of research design and so the 12 included studies ranged from systematic reviews and randomized controlled trials to anecdotal studies.

Steultjens et al. (2005) also had general criteria. Their two inclusion criteria were that the review evaluated the efficacy of OT intervention and that the review was a systematic search, including electronic search, of research over a specified time period. The only exclusion criteria were reviews of multidisciplinary interventions or interventions by other healthcare disciplines.

The criteria used by Steultjens et al. (2004) were more detailed, and included:

Type of study – RCTs, CCTs and other designs (which included pre-post test designs and case series studies)
Participants – diagnosis of rheumatoid arthritis
Intervention – six interventions were identified:

■ training of motor function
■ training of skills
■ instruction on joint protection
■ counselling
■ advice on the use of assistive devices
■ provision of splints

Outcomes – included measures of:

■ pain
■ fatigue
■ function
■ independence
■ quality of life
■ knowledge of disease management

The selection process to decide whether studies met the inclusion criteria was carried out by three members of the research team.

protocol should ensure that bias is reduced by explicitly outlining the inclusion and exclusion criteria. The use of methodological quality criteria also ensures the rigour of the review and the inclusion of high-quality research evidence, thus ensuring that any conclusions are based on the strongest available research evidence.

Using the inclusion/exclusion criteria, studies should then be selected or rejected. This process should be carried out by more than one reviewer, to reduce bias. All excluded trials should be listed within the review, with the reasons for exclusion outlined. Of the initial 31 publications identified by Barras (2005) only 12 met the inclusion criteria. In the Cochrane review of OT for rheumatoid arthritis

Box 4.4 Quality assessment

The process of quality assessment within Cochrane Reviews is clearly defined. Steultjens *et al.* (2004) used the tool developed by Van Tulder *et al.* (1997), which consists of 19 criteria covering internal validity, descriptive and statistical criteria. The tool was adapted slightly for the studies in the category 'other designs' and the quality assessment process was conducted by two of the researchers independently.

Barras (2005) used three scales to assess methodological quality. The McMaster Scales (Law *et al.* 1998) were used, as appropriate, for the quantitative and qualitative papers, and the READER Critical Appraisal Method (MacAuley & McGram 1999) was used for all papers. It is interesting to note that all quantitative studies were assessed using the same tool, although the review included both systematic reviews and RCTs, which should arguably be assessed using different criteria.

Steultjens *et al.* (2005) made no attempt to assess or comment on the methodological quality of the systematic reviews included in their review of reviews.

by Steultjens *et al.* (2004), 43 papers of the original 2694 citations fulfilled all of the inclusion criteria for the review. In the review of reviews by Steultjens *et al.* (2005), of the 581 potential reviews only 14 met the inclusion criteria.

The methodological quality of the included studies is then assessed (Box 4.4). A variety of tools have been developed for the assessment of methodological quality, particularly of RCTs (e.g. Jadad *et al.* 1996; Van Tulder *et al.* 1997; Maher 2003). Agreement on the assessment of the methodological quality of qualitative research is more complex and fewer assessment tools have been developed (the issue of methodological quality in qualitative research will be discussed in more depth in Chapter 5).

Having identified and assessed the relevant and appropriate studies, the next stage is to extract and synthesize the relevant data from each of the research papers to be included in the review. Various methods of data synthesis are available to the systematic reviewer. However, it is not the task of this chapter to review these methods (more details on this process are discussed in Chapter 8). The outcomes of data synthesis will be discussed in the next section of this chapter (Understanding the numbers in systematic reviews) and also in more detail in Chapter 8. The final stage of the systematic review process is to interpret the findings, drawing in all the available evidence, assessing the strength of the evidence and evaluating the effectiveness of the intervention under review.

Whilst systematic reviews aim to provide the least biased and most reliable summary of available evidence, they are not without their limitations. The main areas of limitation and bias in systematic reviews are publication bias, study quality and the diversity of studies. Publication bias, and the tendency to publish only interesting and positive results, has already been mentioned in the discussion of RCTs in Chapter 3. Systematic reviews endeavour to overcome publication bias

> **Box 4.5** Similarity and diversity of included studies
>
> One of the purposes of systematic reviews is to provide some form of synthesis of the findings from the various studies within the review. However, if the studies are too dissimilar this can prove impossible.
>
> Barras (2005) included a number of different methodological types of study (systematic reviews, RCTs and descriptive studies). She also noted that a wide range of outcomes were measured including falls, ability to cope and quality of life. Thus, because of the diversity of methodologies and outcomes, the only synthesis that was possible was the use of summary tables and narrative.
>
> Within a Cochrane review a greater level of homogeneity (similarity) might be expected. However, the review of Steultjens *et al.* (2004) acknowledged that there was a considerable degree of heterogeneity (diversity) amongst the studies, particularly in terms of participants (due to varying levels of disease severity), intervention (in terms of duration, frequency and setting even when similar interventions were studied) and a diversity of outcome measures.
>
> Given the diversity of patient groups included in the review of reviews by Steultjens *et al.* (2005), ranging from children with cerebral palsy, through people with mental health problems to older people, and the range of types of study within each of the reviews, there is a considerable level of heterogeneity within this review.

by accessing information from unpublished sources, theses and conferences where neutral or nonsignificant findings may be discussed.

Systematic reviews are only as good as the primary data they reanalyse. Not all systematic reviews are rigorous about the methodological quality criteria used to include and exclude studies. A famous criticism of systematic reviews was proposed by Eysenck (1978, p. 517)

> a mass of reports – good, bad, and indifferent – are fed into the computer . . . 'garbage in – garbage out'.

Interestingly, both Cusick (1986) and de Vet *et al.* (1997) argue that the inclusion of poor-quality studies need not affect the outcome of a meta-analysis.

Diversity is the final area of limitation and potential bias in systematic reviews (Box 4.5). The nature of systematic reviews is that the results of a number of studies are compared. However, the similarities and diversity of the various studies must be considered in terms of the following questions:

■ How similar are the participants in each study?
■ What is the context of the various trials?
■ Can studies from different countries be compared?
■ Can studies of inpatient and outpatient settings and interventions be compared?
■ How comparable are the various interventions?

It might be possible to justify the homogeneity (similarity) of the various study populations or, if there is evidence of heterogeneity (differences), it might be necessary to compare subgroups within the populations or to take the hetero-geneity into account in the data analysis.

Understanding the numbers in systematic reviews

The main task of any meta-analysis is to take each trial and compare the number of participants in the intervention group who had a successful outcome with the number of participants in the control group who had a successful outcome. The comparisons can then be totalled to give an overall *effects score*. However, the analysis is not quite as simple as this makes it sound. It is often impossible to cal-culate a simple comparison because the numbers of participants in the interven-tion group and the control group vary. The comparison is, therefore, usually expressed in terms of an *odds ratio* (Langhorne & Dennis 1998; Pereira-Maxwell 1998). Although, as Box 4.6 illustrates, other measures are also used in meta-analysis.

An odds ratio is a number that expresses the ratio of the likelihood (odds) of a particular outcome (e.g. improved function, death, level of independence) occur-ring amongst the participants in the intervention group in comparison with the likelihood (odds) of that outcome occurring in the control group. It should be noted that, somewhat perversely, odds ratios are usually expressed in terms of the prevention of a bad outcome (e.g. death, dependence) rather than in terms of a positive outcome (e.g. improved function). An *odds ratio of 1* indicates that there

---

Box 4.6 Meta-analysis and other forms of data synthesis

Because the reviews of both Barras (2005) and Steultjens *et al.* (2005) had high levels of het-erogeneity the analysis and synthesis were based solely on summary tables and a narrative synthesis.

Because of the diversity of the studies and their relatively poor methodological quality, Barras (2005) concluded that there was some evidence that OT home assessments form an integral aspect of patient care and that they have some effect on quality of life, number of falls and patient autonomy. However, there is no conclusive evidence of the effectiveness of OT home assessments within discharge planning, mainly because there is too little research to support any conclusions. Whilst Steultjens *et al.* (2005) concluded that although there was only sparse evidence for the effectiveness of specific OT interventions there was evidence to indicate that both older people and people with rheumatoid arthritis and following a stroke would benefit from comprehensive OT intervention.

Steultjens *et al.* (2004) acknowledged that due to the heterogeneity of the studies a meta-analysis was not possible. However, they were able to calculate odds ratios or mean differences (with 95% confidence intervals) for the various studies and to perform a best evidence syn-thesis. They concluded that there is strong evidence for the efficacy of the provision of joint protection information, that limited evidence exists for the use of comprehensive OT interven-tions to improve functional ability and that there are indications that splinting reduces pain.

is the same likelihood (odds) of the outcome occurring in both the intervention and the control groups. An odds ratio of *less than 1* indicates a better outcome in the intervention group, or evidence for the effectiveness of the intervention. An odds ratio of *more than 1* indicates better outcomes in the control group, or no evidence for the effectiveness of the intervention. Odds ratios are always shown with a confidence interval (CI), usually of 95% (see Chapter 3 for a discussion of confidence intervals). A confidence interval is included because the odds ratio is not an accurate estimate of the 'true' value for the population and so a 95% CI gives the best estimation of the possible range of odds.

The results of a meta-analysis are usually presented in a table format, where the results of each trial are presented and the overall total is given at the bottom of the table. Figure 4.1 is an example of meta-analysis results from a review by Langhorne and Dennis (1998) of the effectiveness of stroke units. Because of the number of black squares or dots (blobs) in the table, these tables are often referred to as *blobbograms*.

Comparison:	Organised stroke unit care vs conventional care			
Outcome:	Death or dependency by the end of scheduled follow-up			
Study	Expt n/N	Ctrl n/N	OR (95%CI Fixed)	OR (95%CI Fixed)
Birmingham	8/29	9/23		0.59 [0.18, 1.91]
Dover	65/116	79/117		0.61 [0.36, 1.04]
Edinburgh	93/155	94/156		0.99 [0.63, 1.56]
Helsinki	47/121	65/122		0.56 [0.33, 0.93]
Illinois	20/56	17/35		0.59 [0.25, 1.39]
Kuopio	31/50	31/45		0.74 [0.31, 1.73]
Montreal	58/65	60/65		0.69 [0.21, 2.30]
New York	23/42	23/40		0.89 [0.37, 2.14]
Newcastle	26/34	28/33		0.58 [0.17, 2.00]
Nottingham	123/176	100/139		0.91 [0.55, 1.48]
Orpington (1993)	101/124	108/121		0.53 [0.25, 1.10]
Orpington (1995)	34/34	37/37		0.92 [0.02, 47.65]
Perth	10/29	14/30		0.60 [0.21, 1.72]
Tampere	53/98	55/113		1.24 [0.72, 2.14]
Trondheim	54/110	81/110		0.35 [0.20, 0.61]
Umeå	52/110	102/183		0.71 [0.44, 1.14]
Uppsala	45/60	41/52		0.80 [0.33, 1.95]
Total (95%CI)	**843/1409**	**944/1421**		**0.71 [0.60, 0.84]**

Figure 4.1 Example of meta-analysis results. For an explanation of abbreviations see text. Meta-analysis comparing stroke unit care with conventional care: death or dependency at the end of follow-up (median 1 year: range 6 weeks to 1 year). (Reproduced with permission from Langhorne, P. & Dennis, M. (1998) *Stroke Units: An Evidence Based Approach*. London: BMJ Publishing Group, p. 44.)

The blob (or black square) represents the odds ratio for the particular trial and the horizontal line represents the 95% confidence interval for that odds ratio. This line is often referred to as the *wobble factor*, as it represents the uncertainty and possible variation of the odds ratio. The vertical line down the table is known as *the line of no effect*, and represents an odds ratio of 1. Thus, trials with a blob to the right of the vertical line (e.g. Tampere in Fig. 4.1) indicate a more favourable outcome in the control group. Trials where the potential (wobble) outcome (e.g. Birmingham in Fig. 4.1), as indicated by the 95%CI, *might* be in favour of the control group are shown with a confidence interval line that crosses the line of no effect.

In Fig. 4.1 the information given in the table includes:

- the name of the study;
- the number of participants in the intervention group (Expt) with an adverse result (*n*) in comparison with the total number of participants in the intervention group (*N*);
- corresponding data for the control group (Ctrl);
- graphic representation of the odds ratio (OR) and 95% confidence interval (95%CI);
- the actual numerical data for the odds ratio and 95%CI.

At the bottom of the table is the total result for the review represented with a diamond. The centre of the diamond is the total odds ratio and the width of the diamond shows the 95% confidence interval for the total odds ratio.

According to Fig. 4.1, the Montreal study had 65 participants in both the intervention and control groups. Of the 65 patients treated on a stroke unit (the experimental group) 58 were either dead or dependent – as opposed to independent, measured on an Activities of Daily Living (ADL) score – by the end of the follow-up period. Of the 65 patients who were treated on a conventional care ward 60 were dead or dependent by the end of the follow-up. When converted this gives an odds ratio of 0.69, which is in favour of the intervention, and a 95% confidence interval of odds ratios from 0.21 to 2.30, indicating a degree of wobble from favouring stroke unit care to favouring conventional care. The total results, however, favour stroke units, with a total odds ratio of 0.71 and a 95% confidence interval from 0.60 to 0.84; all of these values are on the intervention side of the line of no effect. From these findings it might be safe to conclude that stroke units are effective not only in preventing death but also in reducing the level of dependence.

For the client-centred evidence-based occupational therapist the use of research evidence to inform intervention decisions must be explicit, judicious and conscientious (to paraphrase Sackett's definition of evidence-based medicine; see Chapter 1). However, faced with the findings of a meta-analysis how does the therapist share this confusing and daunting information with her client? Tickle-Degnen (1998) points out that the therapist must be able to translate the quantitative information into meaningful clinical information, in terms of the likelihood that an intervention might be successful or useful for that particular client. This is where the appraisal skills of the evidence-based occupational therapist are important.

Appraising systematic reviews

As with any appraisal, the appraisal of a systematic review addresses the three main questions:

- Are the results valid?
- What are the results?
- How will these results help me work with my clients?

Table 4.1 gives an overview of the questions to ask when appraising a systematic review. These questions are based on the questions developed as part of the Critical Appraisal Skills Programme (CASP) initiative with some additions, which the author felt were relevant to evidence-based OT (see Chapter 10 for more information about the CASP programme).[1]

Table 4.1 Questions to ask when critically appraising a systematic review.

Are the results valid?
- Did the review address a clearly focused issue?
- Do you think the important, relevant studies were included?
- Did the reviewers establish clear inclusion and exclusion criteria for the identified studies?
- Did the review's authors do enough to assess the methodological quality of the included studies?
- If the results of the review have been combined, was it reasonable to do so?

What are the results?
- If a meta-analysis and synthesis was used, were the methods of meta-analysis appropriate and clearly justified?
- What is the overall result of the review?
- How precise are the results?
- Are the conclusions and recommendations based on the review findings?

How will these results help me work with my clients?
- Can the results be applied to the local population of my practice and clients?
- Were all important outcomes considered?
- Are the benefits worth the harms and costs?

---

[1] Other examples of appraisal checklists for systematic reviews can be found at: CASP (http://www.phru.nhs.uk/casp/critical_appraisal_tools.htm#s/reviews);HealthEvidence Bulletins (Wales) (http://hebw.uwcm.ac.uk/methodology/appendix5.htm); Centre for EB Mental Health (http://www.psychiatry.ox.ac.uk/cebmh/education_critical_appraisal.htm).

The reader will note that there are similarities in the questions asked to appraise any piece of research, be it an RCT, a qualitative study or a systematic review. The various questions will now be expanded, within the context of appraising a systematic review. Table 4.2 contains a worked example of a critical appraisal of a systematic review (Tse 2005).

Are the results valid?

Did the review address a clearly focused issue?

As with the appraisal of RCTs or qualitative research, the first question to ask when appraising a systematic review is whether the review has a clear aim and research question. If the aim is broad, have the reviewers asked smaller, subsidiary questions? Did the reviewers clearly establish the parameters of the review question in terms of the population to be included, the interventions to be reviewed and compared, and the outcomes being measured?

This question can be used as a screening process to help you decide whether it is worth spending precious reading time on a particular review. If the answers to this question are negative it is probably not worth continuing to read and appraise the review, as it will provide poor-quality evidence of effectiveness.

Do you think the important, relevant studies were included?

As we have seen, studies need to be gathered from a range of sources. Have the reviewers given full details of the search strategy, including the key words used? Were these adequate and appropriate to the topic? Have the reviewers searched a range of databases? Knowing that not all research is published, have the reviewers made efforts to find unpublished research? Have the reviewers followed up reference lists and contacted experts and specialists in the appropriate fields?

Did the reviewers establish clear inclusion and exclusion criteria for identified studies?

Having identified relevant studies, how did the reviewers approach the task of deciding which studies to include or exclude from the review? Did the reviewers outline the criteria they used? To avoid bias, was more than one person involved in inclusion/exclusion decisions? Have details of excluded studies and the reasons for exclusion been given? It is also worth considering the nature of the inclusion and exclusion criteria. Have the reviewers been too narrow or too broad in their criteria? If there is a cut-off date for the search is it too recent to include all relevant studies? Has the study focused on English language papers or on published papers only – again this might miss relevant non-English or unpublished research. What types of research have been included within the review? Might it have been valuable to include studies outside the narrow clinical trials methodology?

Table 4.2 Worked example of a critical appraisal of a systematic review: Tse, T. (2005) The environment and falls prevention: do environmental modifications make a difference? *Australian Occupational Therapy Journal* **52**, 271–281.

Question	Yes, no, can't tell	Comments
Are the results valid?		
Screening question: Did the review address a clearly focused issue?	Yes	The review does appear to have a clear focus:
		To review the literature, no more than 15 years old, and to present a comprehensive summary of effective environmental modification strategies.
		Falls prevention is currently a 'hot topic' within the care of older people and Tse, in her introduction, points out that the links between environmental modifications (such as removing loose mats, changing lighting or installing grab rails) and falls reduction have been contentious. However, there appears to be recent evidence to suggest that environmental modification within multifactorial falls programmes might be effective. The review's goal is to provide evidence to support the role of environmental modification within falls prevention strategies, although this goal may appear to be, in itself, somewhat biased in favour of the value of environmental modifications.

If the answer to this screening question is 'yes', it is worth carrying on with the appraisal?

Question	Yes, no, can't tell	Comments
Do you think the important, relevant studies were included?	Yes	The published literature was extensively searched, using CINAHL, MEDLINE and the Cochrane Database of Systematic Reviews, using an appropriate range of key words. The references included in all potentially useful articles were also scanned for additional studies.
		However, no attempt was made to search the grey literature, which could mean that potentially useful studies were not accessed and, whilst the Cochrane Database of Systematic Reviews was searched it does not appear that either DARE (Database of Abstracts of Reviews of Effectiveness) or the Cochrane Controlled Trials Register, which form part of the Cochrane Library databases, were searched.

(Continued)

Table 4.2 *Continued.*

Question	Yes, no, can't tell	Comments
Did the reviewers establish clear inclusion and exclusion criteria for the identified studies?	Yes/no	A number of inclusion criteria appear to have been used: ▪ Publication between 1994 and 2004 – although the studies within the review include one paper published in 1990 and another published in 1993 ▪ A range of types of research (RCTs, longitudinal studies, reviews) ▪ Participants in the studies must be older people (age limits undefined), not necessarily with a history of falls ▪ Two key outcomes were mentioned – a change in the risk of falling and the prevalence of environmental modifications – but no specific outcome measures were identified. How these various criteria were actually operationalized is unclear and no specific inclusion and exclusion criteria were stated. Eighteen studies were identified for inclusion in the review, but no mention is made of the number of excluded studies or the reasons for any exclusions. It is not clear whether more than one of the authors was involved in the inclusion/exclusion screening. Therefore inclusion/exclusion bias cannot be completely ruled out.
Did the review's authors do enough to assess the methodological quality of the included studies?	Yes/no	Whilst a table (Table 1) provides an overview of the methodological criteria for the 18 included studies, it is unclear how the criteria identified to assess methodological quality were chosen. The six criteria are: ▪ Allocation concealment, which also appears to have been conflated with randomization ▪ Outcome assessor blinded ▪ Subjects comparable at the start ▪ Subjects blinded ▪ Outcome measures defined ▪ Duration.

Table 4.2 *Continued.*

Question	Yes, no, can't tell	Comments
		Given the potential inclusion of a range of types of research the value of a single assessment of methodological quality might be questioned. In fact the majority (16) of the included studies appear to be RCTs, so the review might have been more valuable if it had focused solely on RCTs and used an RCT-specific assessment of methodological quality such as the PEDro scale. There is no mention of more than one person being involved in the quality assessment process. Therefore, given the potential flaws and biases within the quality assessment process, the actually assessment of methodological quality within this review appears to be somewhat limited.
If the results of the review have been combined, was it reasonable to do so?	N/A	The findings of the review were summarized in table form (Table 2 for studies in institutional settings and Table 3 for studies within community settings). Given the heterogeneity of both the participants and the interventions any form of synthesis of the findings would not be possible.
What are the results?		
Were the methods of meta-analysis and synthesis appropriate and clearly justified?	N/A	As stated above synthesis of the findings of the various studies was not appropriate and was not carried out. The findings of the review were presented in narrative form.
What is the overall result of the review?	N/A	Narrative summaries of the various studies with overall comparisons of the findings are presented, divided according to the setting of the studies (institutional or community). Few of the studies appear to have achieved statistically significant results and the only results presented are in percentage form. A number of the included studies appear to be of multifactorial interventions rather than solely focused on environmental modification, so teasing out the actual evidence for the effectiveness of environmental modification in either institutional or community settings is difficult.

(Continued)

Table 4.2 *Continued.*

Question	Yes, no, can't tell	Comments
How precise are the results?	N/A	As mentioned above little statistical evidence is given for the individual studies and no overall synthesis was carried out. It is, therefore, impossible to conclude whether there is any high-quality evidence for the effectiveness of environmental modifications within falls prevention.
Are the conclusions and recommendations based on the review findings?	Yes/no	Tse includes a section on the implications for occupational therapists, which explores a range of issues pertinent to OT intervention in falls prevention programmes and lists six factors that should be included within an OT falls practice; however, none of these factors appears to be based on the evidence discussed within the review. The review concluded that: There is now *some* [emphasis added] evidence that indicates environmental modifications can make a difference for older people with a history of falls and when implemented with other multifactorial interventions. However, the review also concludes that more research is needed.
How will these results help me work with my clients?		*The answers to these questions can only be given by you, the reader, in relation to your service. These are my reflections only.*
Can the results be applied to the local population of my practice and clients?		The review includes evidence from both institutional and community settings with participants some of whom have a history of falls, whilst others have no history of falls. Participants in the included studies are described as 'older' but no clear information is given on the range of ages. There may be appropriate and relevant evidence within this review for occupational therapists working within falls prevention programmes, but the reader will have to work to extract the information that is specifically relevant.

Table 4.2 *Continued.*

Question	Yes, no, can't tell	Comments
Were all important outcomes considered?		The outcomes considered appear to be number of falls and number of injuries; however, there appear to be no standardized tools, which is one of the problems for research in this area.
Are the benefits worth the harms and costs?		The paper does not specifically mention any of these factors, although the costs of equipment in institutional settings and personal factors such as perceived risk and compliance are mentioned briefly as factors to be considered within community settings.

Did the review's authors do enough to assess the methodological quality of the included studies?

As well as giving criteria for inclusion and exclusion, the reviewers should also outline the criteria used for appraising the quality of the research to be included in the review. What quality criteria were used? Were the criteria based on recognized scales such as the PEDro scale, which evidence shows has utility and validity for assessing the quality of clinical trials (Maher 2003)? There is little value in reviewing poor-quality or flawed research evidence. The task of appraising the methodological quality should, like inclusion and exclusion, be a shared task with more than one reviewer independently appraising the methodological rigour of the various papers.

If the results of the review have been combined, was it reasonable to do so?

The characteristics of the various included studies should be presented, probably in table format, to allow you to judge whether the studies are similar enough to allow comparisons to be made. Were the study designs similar? Were the interventions similar? Have similar outcome measures been used? If there is evidence of heterogeneity, has this been accounted for in the statistical analysis?

What are the results?

Were the methods of meta-analysis and synthesis appropriate and clearly justified?

Various methods are used for meta-analysis. Has the process of data extraction and analysis been clearly explained and justified? Do the methods used appear to be appropriate for the various studies and types of data?

What is the overall result of the review?

Does the overall result of the review address the research question? If the review asked subsidiary questions, have these been answered by the results? Have overall results been given for the various outcome measures? Has the statistical significance of any differences between interventions been tested? Have measures of clinical significance been used?

How precise are the results?

Have results been presented with confidence intervals? Is the confidence interval used (e.g. 90%, 95%) appropriate?

Are the conclusions and recommendations based on the review findings?

Sometime reviews become overenthusiastic about the nature and strength of the findings of their review, and the conclusions and recommendations go beyond what could reasonably be concluded from the actual findings. Look carefully at the conclusions and the recommendations. Are they based on the findings of high-quality research evidence? Are they based on the findings of the review or have the authors included their own ideas and assumptions?

How will these results help me work with my clients?

Can the results be applied to the local population of my practice and clients?

Consider the nature of the population covered by the reviewed trials; how similar is it to your client group? Can the findings be applied to your particular setting? Are the review population and your client group similar enough?

Were all important outcomes considered?

A review is only as broad as its original parameters; some outcomes will not be assessed. However, does the review cover all the outcomes you are concerned with?

Are the benefits worth the harms and costs?

The review may include some form of cost/benefit discussion, but if not, what do you think? Is the strength of the intervention worth any possible costs or harms?

Gray (2001) argues that systematic reviews are the best source of evidence for healthcare decision- and policy-makers. However, he does add the note of caution that the quality of systematic reviews is variable. Any systematic review should be appraised carefully before any judgments are made.

Activity

▩ Identify a systematic review of relevance to your area of practice/interest.
▩ Using the appraisal questions above, work with a colleague to appraise the article and to assess its value as evidence.
▩ The Cochrane Library is a major source of information on systematic reviews. Spend some time exploring the Cochrane Library Database of Systematic Reviews.

Further reading

The following references will allow the reader to explore the value and use of systematic reviews and meta-analyses in more depth.

Chalmers, I. & Altman, D.G. (eds) (1995) *Systematic Reviews*. London: BMJ Publishing Group.

Cusick, A. (1986) Research in occupational therapy: meta-analysis. *Australian Occupational Therapy Journal* **33**(4), 142–147.

Green, S. & Higgins, J. (eds) (2005) *Cochrane Handbook for Systematic Reviews of Interventions 4.2.5* [updated May 2005] (http://www.cochrane.uk/cochrane/handbook/handbook.htm) [accessed 18 June 2006].

Greenhalgh, T. (2006) *How to Read a Paper*, 3rd edn. Oxford: Blackwell Publishing.

Hayes, R.L. (1998) Evidence-based practice: the Cochrane Collaboration, and occupational therapy. *Canadian Journal of Occupational Therapy* **65**(3), 144–151.

Langhorne, P. & Dennis, M. (1998) *Stroke Units: an Evidence Based Approach*. London: BMJ Publishing Group.

McKinnell, I. & Elliott, J. (1997) *The Cochrane Library: Self-Training Guide & Notes*. Oxford: NHS Executive Anglia & Oxford.

Mulrow, C.D. (1994) Rationale for systematic reviews. *British Medical Journal* **309**, 597–599.

Petticrew, M. & Roberts, H. (2006) *Systematic Reviews in the Social Sciences*. Oxford: Blackwell Publishing.

Sinclair, A. & Dickinson, E. (1998) *Effective Practice in Rehabilitation*. London: King's Fund.

Tickle-Degnen, L. (1998) Communicating with clients about treatment outcomes: the use of meta-analytic evidence in collaborative treatment planning. *American Journal of Occupational Therapy* **52**(7), 526–530.

5: Qualitative research as evidence

Qualitative research has, for some time, been seen as the methodology of choice for occupational therapy (OT) research (Kielhofner 1982; Krefting 1989a; Yerxa 1991). The results of a quick search of both CINAHL and AMED are summarized in Table 5.1. Two things are particularly noteworthy here: the value of using a variety of search terms (i.e. not just qualitative research but the various approaches within qualitative research) and also the apparent superiority of CINAHL.

Qualitative research has, until recently, had a less prominent place in evidence-based practice. Qualitative research is often, albeit wrongly, viewed as lacking validity and reliability. Numbers, and anything that can be quantified, are acceptable as 'scientific' facts and, therefore, as evidence. Ideas, as mere words, are seen as biased and unscientific and, therefore, of limited value as evidence. As Greenhalgh (2006) points out, even 'facts' that have little evidence to support them are accepted because of the apparent evidence of the numbers.

Qualitative research is beginning to be seen as acceptable and appropriate as evidence to answer certain questions. More and more healthcare researchers are realizing that RCTs do not answer all the relevant questions. Qualitative research generates deeper, richer data, which can address issues of quality and the client's experience of healthcare. In the previous chapter on systematic reviews, we saw how stroke units can be effective in reducing disability. What this research cannot tell us is why stroke units are more effective than other, equally rehabilitation-orientated, medical units.

Qualitative research can have a number of uses within the context of evidence-based practice (EBP). Morse *et al.* (1998) have shown how qualitative research can be used to develop clinical assessment guides. Further, Kearney (2001) has argued that qualitative studies, which explore the experience of illness or disability, can be used as aides to guiding and coaching patients who might be experiencing similar problems and issues. Qualitative research can also aid our understanding of the real clinical value of the findings of quantitative studies (Barbour 2000). The use of narratives based on experience can also challenge and develop our understanding of particular experiences or phenomena by making us think more deeply or presenting us with different ways of seeing the world.

Working groups within both the Cochrane and Campbell Collaborations (Cochrane Qualitative Research Methods Group; Campbell Implementation

Table 5.1 Searching for occupational therapy qualitative research: numbers of hits corresponding to various combinations of key words.

	AMED	CINAHL
Qualitative research AND occupational therapy	53	211
Phenomenology AND occupational therapy	5	51
Ethnography AND occupational therapy	14	44
Grounded theory AND occupational therapy	28	65
Qualitative research OR phenomenology OR ethnography OR grounded theory AND occupational therapy	95	327

Process Methods Group: http://www.joannabriggs.edu.au/cqrmg/about.html) are currently developing criteria for appraising qualitative research and using qualitative research within systematic reviews (Popay & Williams 1998; Petticrew & Roberts 2006). Qualitative research has played a major role in OT for some time, and is now beginning to be seen as an important and valuable source of evidence within healthcare. The evidence-based occupational therapist should find qualitative research a rich source of valuable evidence and reflection on her or his interventions and practice.

This chapter will give a brief overview of research from a qualitative perspective, beginning by outlining the methodology, approaches and methods of qualitative research. The chapter will then explore the often contentious issue of how qualitative research can be seen as 'good' research. The chapter concludes with an overview of how the evidence-based occupational therapist can appraise qualitative research as evidence for the effectiveness of interventions and practice. As with the previous two chapters, examples of 'real' OT research will be used to illustrate various points.

Overview of qualitative research

Research is often seen as being divided into two *methodologies* or philosophical paradigms. These differing, and for some opposing, methodologies are qualitative research and quantitative research. Once the research methodology is identified, all research can then be divided into particular research *approaches*. In quantitative research the approaches include:

▪ experiments
▪ randomized controlled trials (RCTs)
▪ surveys

In qualitative research the approaches include:

▪ phenomenology
▪ ethnography
▪ grounded theory

Within any research approach a variety of research *methods* can be used to gather the actual data for the study. These research methods include:

■ measurement
■ observation
■ interviews
■ diaries

Qualitative methodology

Qualitative and quantitative research are often seen as diametrically opposed (DePoy & Gitlin 2005). But although qualitative and quantitative research are based on radically different philosophical paradigms, both methodologies are ways of viewing the process of empirical investigation. Table 5.2 summarizes the differences between the two methodologies (Krefting 1989a; Bailey 1997; DePoy & Gitlin 2005; Greenhalgh 2006).

Table 5.2 Overview of the differences between qualitative and quantitative methodology.

	Qualitative methodology	Quantitative methodology
Philosophical background	Realism/existentialism	Rationalism/positivism
Philosophical approach	Holistic	Reductionist
Academic fields	Sociology, anthropology, social psychology	Natural sciences, medicine, psychology
Reasoning	Inductive	Deductive
Mode of enquiry	Naturalistic enquiry	Scientific method
Perspective	Emic (insider) Subjective	Etic (outsider) Objective
Research question	Explores a research question Describes and understands a setting or phenomenon	Tests a hypothesis Demonstrates cause and effect
Research process	Researcher is inside the research setting Definitions evolve with the research Flexible approach	Researcher stands outside the research setting Specific operational definitions are established Control Clearly defined process
Data	Words Subjective Observations, interviews Content analysis	Numbers Measurement Objective Statistical analysis
Rigour	Trustworthiness	Validity and reliability

Box 5.1 Aims and questions in qualitative studies

Woodside *et al.* (2006) used a qualitative approach to gain a better understanding of the insights regarding vocational success of people who had experienced at least one episode of psychosis. The study did not state a research question as such but its purpose was to suggest factors contributing to vocational success.

Chard (2006) explored the experiences of a group of occupational therapists following a continuing professional development course on the use of the Assessment of Motor and Process Skills (AMPS). The aim of the study was to explore the occupational therapists' experiences and the challenges and barriers they faced when attempting to adopt AMPS within their existing professional practice.

In the study of Sellar and Boshoff (2006) the aim was to explore the leisure experiences of well older people. Their research question was 'what are the leisure experiences of retired older Australians living independently in the community?'

Goodacre (2006) carried out a longitudinal qualitative study, over two years, to gain a greater understanding of the impact of chronic arthritis on the lives of women. She wanted to explore the strategies the women used to minimize the impact of the disease on activity and how these strategies were integrated into their lives.

The aim of quantitative research in healthcare (RCTs, systematic reviews) is to provide statistical evidence to evaluate the effectiveness of particular interventions. By contrast, the aim of qualitative research is to explore phenomena in their natural settings, to explore the meanings and interpretations people bring to their everyday lives and experiences, and to explore the complexities of human life and behaviour (Denzin & Lincoln 1994) (Box 5.1). Quantitative research can often strip the context and the humanity away from the focus and setting of the research. For qualitative research, context is vitally important. In health and social care terms, qualitative research can address such questions as:

- What stops people giving up smoking? (Greenhalgh 2006)
- What is it like to live with the aftermath of traumatic head injury? (Krefting 1989b)
- What makes any activity meaningful? (Taylor & McGruder 1996)

Qualitative research approaches

Qualitative research can be used to 'understand the meanings, experiences, and phenomena as they evolve in the natural setting' (DePoy & Gitlin 2005, p. 48). This can be done from a variety of different perspectives, by asking different types of research questions. The different perspectives and research questions will need to be explored using different research approaches.

Ethnography aims to describe a culture (Krefting 1989a; Bailey 1997; DePoy & Gitlin 2005). Ethnography has been used within anthropology to describe and interpret cultural patterns of groups, to understand cultural meanings and to understand how people organize and interpret their experience. The sorts of research questions asked in ethnographic studies are, broadly, 'what is happening here and why is it happening?' (Box 5.2).

Box 5.2 Example of ethnographic studies relevant to OT

Townsend's (1996) study of mental health OT practice posed the question 'what are the possibilities and constraints for occupational therapists to enable the empowerment of adults who attend mental health day programmes?' She explored this issue using an institutional ethnographic process.

The study of Spencer *et al.* (1995) observed the life of a patient following spinal cord injury and how he learnt the culture of rehabilitation and of being a disabled person.

Box 5.3 Examples of phenomenological studies relevant to OT

Missiuna *et al.* (2006) utilized a phenomenological approach to explore the experiences of parents of children who had been diagnosed with developmental coordination disorder (DCD). Parents of children with DCD were purposefully sampled to ensure variation of age, gender and geographical location, and 13 parents participated in the study. Participants were interviewed twice and completed a standardized questionnaire about their child's symptoms and attributes. Three themes emerged from the data, relating to the parents' struggle to understand their child's problems, negotiating interactions with care professionals to access support, and the dilemma of knowing the best way to help their child. Whilst the authors identify practical implications for OT, the key strength of this paper is in providing information to share with parents in terms of the guiding role identified by Kearney (2001).

Finlay's (1997) insightful study of how occupational therapists view their clients revealed how occupational therapists use social evaluations and how clients can be categorized as 'good', 'bad' or 'difficult'.

Kloczko and Ikiugo (2006) conducted a small phenomenological study into the role of OT with adolescents with eating disorders. They interviewed three occupational therapists working with this client group, asking them to describe their role and the models and interventions that they used.

Bailey (1997) proposes that successful ethnography helps the reader to behave appropriately in the particular cultural setting, whether the setting is a mental-health care facility, rehabilitation unit or day-care centre for clients with dementia (Hasselkus 1992).

Phenomenological research aims to explore the lived experience of individuals. Particular phenomena (or events, or experiences) are explored in an attempt to understand how individuals interpret and give meaning to their lives. Whereas ethnography can involve interpretation and critical analysis on the part of the researcher, meaning and interpretation within phenomenology are drawn from the participants. Phenomenological research, therefore, unlike ethnography, cannot be generalized. The insights and understandings of individuals' experience gained from phenomenological research can, however, be used as tools to reflect upon and evaluate practice for the evidence-based occupational therapist (Box 5.3).

Box 5.4 Examples of grounded-theory studies relevant to OT

Whitcher and Tse (2004) used a grounded-theory approach to explore how counselling skills are used in mental health OT. The study consisted of four phases of data collection, in order to develop the data collection tool and to validate the developing findings. Data collection techniques included focus groups, individual interviews and observations of occupational therapists interacting with clients. Findings were used to develop a model to show that occupational therapists in mental-health settings use counselling skills within a context of occupation.

Craik and Rappolt (2003) developed their theory of research utilization enhancement for occupational therapists and their model of research utilization in OT as a result of a grounded-theory study of 11 'elite' occupational therapists working in adult stroke rehabilitation. Data were collected by interviews, observations and analysis of policy documents.

The type of questions asked in phenomenological research might include:

- What is the meaning of independence for a disabled person? (e.g. McCuaig & Frank 1991)
- What is the meaning of rehabilitation for patients following a cerebrovascular accident (CVA)?

The final qualitative approach to be discussed here is *grounded theory* (Box 5.4). The main aim of grounded theory is theory generation. A broad topic area is developed; the researcher then gathers data relevant to the topic using participants who might be seen to have particular knowledge of the topic. The process of data collection is continued until the researcher feels all possible avenues are exhausted. Much of the early clinical reasoning research in OT adopted a grounded-theory approach (Mattingly & Fleming 1994).

Research methods in qualitative research

A variety of *methods* of data collection are used in qualitative research (Box 5.5), the main ones being:

- interviews
- focus groups
- observations
- written materials

Analysis, within qualitative research, is an ongoing process, which takes place throughout the research. Unlike quantitative research, where analysis takes place once data collection is completed, qualitative analysis consists of coding, describing and categorizing the themes that emerge from the research data. A vital tool in this process is the researcher's field log and reflective diary (DePoy & Gitlin 2005).

> **Box 5.5** Methods used in OT qualitative research studies
>
> Woodside *et al.* (2006) used semistructured interviews to explore the occupational experiences and vocational goals of their participants. The interview questions were modified and refined as the study progressed. This study included investigator triangulation, as a number of interviewers were involved in the data collection process.
>
> Each participant in Chard's (2006) study of the use of AMPS was interviewed three times over a 9-month period; the interviews were loosely structured to allow each participant to give a narrative of their experiences. Participants were also asked to keep a reflective journal and the researcher kept a field journal.
>
> Data collection in the study of leisure by Sellar and Boshoff (2006) was by means of an interview. An interview protocol of eight questions was included in the published paper. The interview began by asking participants to describe a 'typical day' and then focused more specifically on leisure experiences.
>
> Goodacre (2006) used a variety of data collection methods in her 2-year study of women's experiences of living with chronic arthritis. Each participant was interviewed twice and took part in a focus group. The interview guide was included as an appendix to the published paper. Each respondent was also asked to keep a 7-day diary, structured into half-hour periods, where the participant recorded her activities throughout the 7-day period; these diaries were used to inform the interviews. The researcher also kept a field diary.

What makes 'good' qualitative research?

One of the problems to have bedevilled qualitative research is the issue of whether qualitative research can be seen as 'good', rigorous research. Frequently, qualitative research is evaluated using validity and reliability criteria that are suitable for quantitative research. Indeed, Mays and Pope (2000) have argued for the use of modified forms of criteria such as validity and relevance to be used as ways of assessing the quality of qualitative research. However, criteria that focus on the generalizability or replicability of research are inappropriate for a methodology that seeks to describe experiences and social complexities (Krefting 1991). This does not mean that qualitative research cannot be evaluated. It means, however, that a different approach must be used. It is important for the evidence-based occupational therapist to understand the ways of ensuring that qualitative research is rigorous, in order for her or him to appraise qualitative research from an appropriate perspective.

Trustworthiness in qualitative research

Krefting (1991) proposed that the notion of trustworthiness should be used when evaluating qualitative research. There are four aspects to trustworthiness and various strategies that the qualitative researcher will use to ensure that her or his research is rigorous. Table 5.3 summarizes the aspects and strategies of trustworthiness. The key components of each aspect will be outlined below, with examples from the OT research.

Table 5.3 Key aspects and strategies of trustworthiness.

Aspect	Strategy
Credibility	Prolonged and varied field experience Reflexivity and reflexive field diary Triangulation Member checking
Transferability	Purposive, theoretical or nominated sample Comparison of sample with demographic data Rich description of the research setting Data saturation
Dependability	Audit Triangulation Negative case analysis Data saturation Peer examination
Confirmability	Audit Triangulation Negative case analysis Collaborative analysis Peer review Member checking Reflexivity

Box 5.6 Strategies for ensuring credibility

Both Goodacre (2006) and Chard (2006) used a range of similar strategies to ensure the credibility of their studies. Both studies involved prolonged engagement, the use of reflexive field diaries and triangulation of methods. Goodacre used repeated interviews, focus groups and respondent diaries, whilst Chard used multiple interviews and respondent diaries. Chard also used member checking to obtain her participants' comments on the veracity of the interview data and findings.

Sellar and Boshoff (2006) report the use of reflexivity by means of a field journal as their sole strategy for ensuring credibility. Woodside *et al.* (2006) reported the use of member checking of the analysis as their strategy for credibility.

Credibility

The credibility of the research assesses whether the research is giving a true picture of the phenomenon being studied, based not on the researcher's expectations and assumptions but on the reality of the participants' experiences. A good test of credibility is whether the descriptions and interpretations of the phenomenon are recognizable to people outside the research setting.

There are various ways of ensuring credibility (Box 5.6). To be able to get a true and detailed picture it is necessary to collect data over a prolonged period of time and from a range of participants. If possible, data should also be collected using a variety of research methods. This process is known as triangulation. However, the length of time and the closeness of contact with participants can result in the researcher finding it difficult to differentiate her/his experiences from those of the participants. This is where a reflexive approach (Finlay 1998) is vitally important. The researcher should keep a field diary to enable reflection and to keep a record of thoughts, feelings, ideas and assumptions as the research progresses. A final strategy for ensuring credibility is to involve participants in the analysis of the research, by giving them access not only to the transcribed data but also to the interpretations and allowing the participants to comment on the research.

Transferability

The second aspect of trustworthiness is whether the research can be seen as transferable to other settings. This can be seen in terms of how well the study achieves 'goodness of fit' with other contexts. However, as Lincoln and Guba (1985) note, transferability is more the responsibility of the reader than the researcher. The researcher's task is to describe the setting in sufficient detail to allow comparisons to be drawn.

The strategies used to ensure transferability focus mainly on the sampling of participants for the study (Box 5.7). The key factor is that the participants are a meaningful representation of the group being studied. This can be done in a variety of ways – by identifying participants who can give meaningful data (purposive sampling); or who allow a theory to be tested (theoretical sampling); or by attempting to match the participants to the demographic variables within the group as a whole; or by using a nominated sample. Nominated sampling is when key informants from the study group identify other people who could be seen as typical of the group.

Box 5.7 Strategies for ensuring transferability

Woodside *et al.* (2006) used purposive sampling to identify potential respondents for their study of vocational success. They had clear eligibility criteria to identify potential participants and gave a demographic overview of the eight participants in a table within the paper.

Sellar and Boshoff (2006) used a detailed screening process to identify their sample of five participants with the capacity to communicate in depth about the concept of leisure. A table gave some information about each participant (e.g. age, living status, health status).

Chard (2006) cited Creswell's (1998) proposal that 20 people should provide sufficient depth of information for a qualitative study. She, therefore, continued recruitment until she had 22 participants. Her participants were occupational therapists, from a wide range of work settings, who had attended an AMPS training course.

Goodacre (2006) gives little information about her sampling strategy apart from her use of local branches of Arthritis Care for access to potential participants. She does, however, give details of her 12 participants in a table (i.e. age, employment, marital status, etc.).

Box 5.8 Strategies for ensuring dependability and confirmability

Chard (2006) employed a comprehensive range of strategies to ensure the dependability and confirmability of her study and its findings. She details the use of reflexivity, member checking audit and the transparency of her research process.

Goodacre (2006) used member checking and a focus group to ensure the trustworthiness of her analysis. She also utilized collaborative analysis, with a colleague reviewing the coding of the transcripts.

Woodside *et al.* (2006) used a number of strategies to ensure the dependability and confirmability of their study. These included reflexivity, member checking and collaborative analysis.

Sellar and Boshoff (2006) mention the use of bracketing, member checking, peer review of the data analysis and reflexivity.

Transferability can also be reviewed in terms of the richness and detail of the background information provided about the participants and the study group. This then allows the reader to assess the goodness of fit to other similar settings.

Dependability

The dependability of a qualitative study relates to how consistent the data and findings are (Box 5.8). In other words, in quantitative terms, how reliable the research is. However, as qualitative research cannot be subject to the same controls as quantitative research, the qualitative researcher can only ensure dependability by clearly explaining the process of the research. This allows the research to be audited and peer reviewed. The researcher enlists the help of colleagues to review the research process.

Confirmability

Confirmability refers to the strategies used by the researcher to limit bias within the research (Box 5.8). In qualitative research this involves the neutrality, not of the researcher, but of the data. The researcher in qualitative research cannot remain outside the research situation. However, she or he can ensure the neutrality of the data by being reflexive and keeping a detailed log of thoughts, ideas and assumptions. The researcher can ask a colleague to audit the research and follow through the decision and analysis process. The researcher can also check ideas and interpretations with participants and expert colleagues.

Appraising qualitative research

Appraisal in general, in particular the development of a checklist approach to the appraisal of qualitative research studies, is hotly debated within both qualitative research and evidence-based practice. Hammersley (1990) and Mays and Pope (2000) have argued that it is possible to identify criteria for the appraisal of qualitative research papers. However, Barbour (2001) has argued strongly that checklists for qualitative research tend to result in a focus on a limited number of technical aspects of qualitative research, such as triangulation or purposive sampling, without a sound understanding or critique of the usefulness of these aspects of qualitative research.

This author contends that it is not possible to established definitive criteria, as it is for quantitative research, but it is possible to establish a number of ground rules that will guide the evidence-based occupational therapist in her or his reading and assessment of qualitative research studies.

As with any appraisal, the appraisal of a qualitative study should address the three main questions:

▥ Are the results trustworthy?
▥ What are the findings?
▥ How will these results help me work with my clients?

Table 5.4 gives an overview of the questions to ask when appraising a qualitative study. These questions are drawn from a range of sources, including Krefting (1991), Greenhalgh (2006) and Gray (2001) and the author's own experience as a qualitative researcher.[1]

Table 5.4 Questions to ask when critically appraising a qualitative study.

Are the results trustworthy?
▥ Was the research question clearly identified?
▥ Was a qualitative methodology and approach appropriate?
▥ Was the setting in which the research took place clearly described?
▥ Were the sampling processes planned, and clearly described?
▥ What was the data collection process and was it clearly described?
▥ What methods were used to analyse the data?
▥ Was the researcher's stance and assumptions clearly articulated and acknowledged?
▥ Were methods used to ensure the credibility of the research?
▥ Did the research workers address issues of confirmability and dependability?
▥ Were ethical issues considered?

What are the findings?
▥ What were the key findings?
▥ Were the results presented in sufficient detail to assess the interpretation of the findings?
▥ What are the conclusions and can they legitimately be drawn from the findings?

How will these results help me work with my clients?
▥ Can the results be applied to my client group and interventions?
▥ Can the study help me in my practice and my interactions with clients?

---

[1] Other examples of appraisal checklists for qualitative studies can be found at: CASP: (http://www.phru.nhs.uk/casp/critical_appraisal_tools.htm#s/reviews); Cochrane Qualitative Research Methods Group: (http://www.joannabriggs.edu.au/cqrmg/tools.html).

The reader will note that there are similarities in the questions asked to appraise any piece of research, be it an RCT, a qualitative study or a systematic review. The various questions will now be expanded, within the context of appraising a qualitative study. Table 5.5 gives a worked example of a critical appraisal of a qualitative study (Wagstaff 2005). The observant reader will notice that there is no middle column for 'Yes/no/can't tell'; this is because it is impossible to make such clear judgments when appraising qualitative research, as the comments in the worked appraisal will illustrate.

Are the results trustworthy?

Was the research question clearly identified?

Although the research question in a qualitative study may be very broad, it is still important for the researchers to outline the aims and objectives of their study, to state a research question, and to give some idea about the parameters of the study.

Was a qualitative methodology and approach appropriate?

What was the study aiming to do? If the focus of the study was an exploration of a phenomenon or to gain an insight into particular issues, then a qualitative methodology is appropriate. Has the researcher identified the research approach used, for instance, ethnography or phenomenology? Is it the most appropriate approach?

Was the setting in which the research took place clearly described?

In terms of the transferability of the study, this is vitally important. The aim of the researcher should be to give the reader sufficient detail about the research setting for the reader to assess the goodness of fit with their own practice setting.

These questions can be used as a screening process to help you to decide whether it is worth spending precious reading time on a particular study. If the answers to these questions are negative it is probably not worth continuing to read and appraise the study, as it will provide poor-quality evidence with limited relevance to practice.

Were the sampling processes planned, and clearly described?

Is the sampling process clearly explained and justified? Did the researcher have clear criteria to identify a suitable purposive sample? Was the researcher attempting to explore a particular theory using a theoretical sample? Did the researcher attempt to make the sample 'representative', either by matching demographic variables or by using a nominated sample? Sampling in qualitative studies can be difficult and researchers often have to resort to convenience or snowball sampling techniques. The researcher might have used the first x (number) people she or he came across, who roughly fitted the study, and this might lead to a biased and unrepresentative sample.

Table 5.5 Worked example of a critical appraisal of a qualitative study: Wagstaff, S. (2005) Supports and barriers for exercise participation for well elders: implications for occupational therapy. *Physical and Occupational Therapy in Geriatrics* **24**(2), 19–33.

Question	Comments
Are the results trustworthy?	
Was the research question clearly identified?	Yes: the focus of the study was the exploration of the perspective of well elderly people of the factors that support or hinder their participation in exercise. A number of sub-questions were identified that linked to the main topic area of the study.
Was a qualitative methodology and approach appropriate?	Yes: the paper argues that the rich data from the older person's perspective are missing from previous research, and the chosen qualitative, phenomenological approach would appear to be the best way of obtaining these data.
Was the setting in which the research took place clearly described?	Yes: purposive sampling was used to identify potential participants. The five participants are clearly described, in pen portraits and a summary table, giving the reader a clear picture of both the research setting and the nature of the sample. The only limitation to transferability is that all five participants are women.
If the answer to these screening questions is 'yes', it is worth carrying on with the appraisal	As the answer to all three screening questions is 'yes' it seems appropriate to continue to appraise this research.
Were the sampling processes planned, and clearly described?	Whilst the sampling strategy is clearly purposive and the sample, whilst small, is appropriate for the study, there would appear to be an element of convenience sampling as the five participants were the five women identified as being both suitable and willing to participate in the study within the chosen research setting. The lack of male participants may also be viewed as a limiting factor. All of the participants took part in some form of exercise at least four times a week; whilst this gives the potential for exploration of factors that facilitate exercise participation it might limit the exploration of factors that inhibit participation.
What was the data collection process and was it clearly described?	Data were collected by means of in-depth interviews with each of the participants. Each interview was guided by a predefined interview protocol. The researcher also kept field notes. Whilst no details of the interview guide are given, the process is adequately described and gives the reader a clear overview of the research process.

Table 5.5 *Continued.*

Question	Comments
What methods were used to analyse the data?	All interviews were transcribed verbatim. The grounded theory analytical approach described by Strauss and Corbin was used to code and categorize the data into emergent themes. The process is clearly described and appears to be appropriate and adequate for the study.
Were the researcher's stance and assumptions clearly articulated and acknowledged?	The researcher's perspective as an occupational therapist is evident, but evidence of reflexivity or the transparency of the researcher's stance and assumptions are lacking.
Were methods used to ensure the credibility of the research?	Although the paper states that 'trustworthiness and credibility of the study were established by the researcher' (p. 24), it is unclear how this was done as there is no mention of member checking or reflexivity, so the credibility of the study could be questioned.
Did the research workers address issues of confirmability and dependability?	There is some evidence of the use of strategies to ensure the dependability and confirmability of the study. Two participants were reinterviewed in order to clarify meanings. Constant comparative analysis and literature triangulation were used in the development of the themes. However, there is no mention of strategies such as data saturation, audit, peer review or reflexivity.
Were ethical issues considered?	Ethics are briefly mentioned in terms of negotiating approval and access with relevant gatekeepers and the use of written consent with each participant, but ethical issues are not discussed in depth.
What are the findings? *What were the key findings?*	Four main themes emerged from the data: ■ Exercise and health – the use of exercise as a way of maintaining health ■ Mental health and vitality – the link between exercise and improved mood and energy levels ■ Mobility and activities of daily living – exercise helps to maintain and improve function ■ Programme design – the importance of access to on-the-spot exercise programmes and facilities. All of the themes present factors that support exercise participation, but there is very little evidence of factors that inhibit or are barriers to exercise participation.

(Continued)

Table 5.5 *Continued.*

Question	Comments
Were the results presented in sufficient detail to assess the interpretation of the findings?	Each theme is illustrated by a number of relevant quotations from the interview data, which give a clear picture of each theme. Aspects of the themes are discussed in the light of previous literature. However, the findings are mostly descriptive and there is little evidence of an interpretative approach to the discussion of the findings.
What are the conclusions and can they legitimately be drawn from the findings?	The findings and discussion are presented together with a separate section covering the implications of the findings for OT. These implications reinforce the value of exercise as a meaningful occupation, which is clearly the key finding from this study.
How will these results help me work with my clients?	*The answers to this question can only really be given by you, the reader, in relation to your service. These are my reflections only.*
Can the results be applied to my client group and interventions?	Whilst these findings have direct relevance to the well elderly population, they may also provide food for thought for occupational therapists working in a range elderly care settings.
Can the study help me in my practice and my interactions with clients?	Exercise has been shown to be a valued occupation and this study provides insight into the factors that might facilitate engagement in exercise activities for older people. However, many people begin exercising and then give up (not just older people) and it might be more meaningful to explore the barriers and inhibitors to exercise participation.

What was the data collection process and was it clearly described?

Data collection in qualitative research is often a long, complex and varied process. The research process in qualitative studies is *iterative* where the researcher may analyse the data alongside the data collection and where the study evolves and changes as it progresses. Have you been given enough information about what the researcher did, and why they chose to do the things they did? If observation was used, was the researcher an active or a passive participant in the setting? If interviews were used, has the researcher given you an overview of the themes and questions? How were the interviews recorded and transcribed? Did the researcher keep a field diary?

What methods were used to analyse the data?

Unlike statistical analysis, the analysis of qualitative data is time-consuming, complex, varied and does not have a standard format. However, has the researcher been systematic in the analysis? You should look out for details of how the data was coded. Is there evidence of *thematic analysis*, or a *constant comparative* approach? Did the researcher *immerse* herself or himself in the data (DePoy & Gitlin 2005)? The use of computer programs to aid qualitative analysis is becoming more common, with programs such as Atlas-ti and NVivo being used to handle large data sets. However, using a computer program to find particular words or phrases can mean that the subtleties within the data set are lost. As Greenhalgh (2006) suggests the VLDRT (very large dining room table) method, where the data are colour coded by felt pen and sorted by cutting and pasting, often produces the highest quality data analysis.

Were the researcher's stance and assumptions clearly articulated and acknowledged?

Qualitative research is based on the premise that reality is subjective and open to individual interpretations. Thus the qualitative researcher is drawing not only on the participants' interpretations but must also acknowledge her or his own perspectives and their influence on the research process. This perspective may be theoretical; for example, my own research is heavily influenced by the theoretical perspectives of the social model of disability. The researcher may also have experiential and tacit knowledge, which has informed the research process. These perspectives need to be acknowledged. Some researchers will argue that they *bracket* their personal knowledge and that this knowledge is put to one side. Many qualitative researchers, however, would argue that bracketing is impossible; what is possible, however, is for the researcher to be transparent and reflexive and to situate themselves (Savin-Baden & Fisher 2002) in relation to the research and the data analysis, so that it is clear where the researcher stands in relation to the study. Reflexivity is crucial in this context.

Were methods used to ensure the credibility of the research?

Strategies for ensuring credibility, discussed above, are prolonged field experience, triangulation, member checking and reflexivity. What evidence is there of these strategies being used in the research? Has the issue of credibility been explored within the study?

Did the research workers address issues of confirmability and dependability?

Was the research process subjected to audit by colleagues of the researcher? Is there sufficient detail in the report to allow you to audit the research? Were the participants involved in reviewing the interpretation of the data? Data that do not fit neatly into the main themes of the analysis comprise an important aspect of any research. How has the researcher dealt with this type of data? Is there evidence of continuing the process of data collection until data saturation has been achieved?

Were ethical issues considered?

By its very nature, qualitative research can be an ethical minefield. Have ethical issues been addressed? Examples include access to participants, procedures for giving informed consent, the confidentiality and anonymity of information and participants, dealing with sensitive issues, and the conflict inherent in being both therapist and researcher.

What are the findings?

What are the key findings?

Results will be presented in terms of themes. Are the themes logical? Are they clearly explained? Do they reflect the aims of the study? Do they help the researcher to answer the research question?

Were the results presented in sufficient detail to assess the interpretation of the findings?

It is important to review how the results were presented. The data of qualitative research are words. The results should include the participants' actual words, rather than summaries of what was said. Where participants are quoted, they should also be identified in some way. Make sure that the full spread of participants' remarks have been quoted, not just one or two people who happened to say what the researcher wanted to hear.

What are the conclusions and can they legitimately be drawn from the findings?

Quantitative research is presented in a standard format of Introduction, Methods, Results, Discussion and Conclusions. It is clear in any quantitative report what the findings (Results) were and how the researcher has interpreted them (Discussion). In qualitative research the results and discussion are often presented together. It is important, therefore, to assess how well the data and the interpretation are linked, whether the interpretation seems logical, and whether it is clear where the interpretation is linked to previous research and also to the researcher's reflexivity. It is important to review the conclusions and to assess how much the conclusions can legitimately be drawn from the study, or whether the researcher is going beyond the data and expressing an unsupported personal opinion.

How will these results help me work with my clients?

Can the results be applied to my client group and interventions?

This question returns to the earlier question of transferability. If the goodness of fit is limited, the research might still give food for thought and evidence for reflection.

Can the study help me in my practice and my interactions with clients?

The potential value of qualitative research to the evidence-based occupational therapist was outlined above. The final question for your appraisal of any paper is 'so what?' What have you learnt from reading this paper? How has this paper challenged or developed your thinking? Will this paper have any value or relevance in your future work?

As Greenhalgh (2006) points out, because qualitative research is becoming more popular and more acceptable there is a danger that poor-quality qualitative research will be published. This is especially true as the tools for evaluating and appraising qualitative research are still being developed. However, as this chapter has shown, qualitative research can be rigorous and it can be appraised. With its focus on the insider perspective, qualitative research should provide the evidence-based occupational therapist with valuable evidence on which to explore the value and effectiveness of client-centred interventions.

▪ ▪

Activity

▪ Identify a qualitative study of relevance to your area of practice/interest.
▪ Using the appraisal questions above, work with a colleague to appraise the article and to assess its value as evidence.

▪ ▪

Further reading

The following references will allow the reader to explore issues pertinent to the design and appraisal of qualitative research in more depth.

Bailey, D.M. (1997) *Research for the Health Professional*, 2nd edn. Philadelphia: FA Davis Co.

Burgess, R. (1984) *In the Field*. London: Unwin Hyman.

Denzin, N.K. & Lincoln, Y.S. (eds) (2005) *Handbook of Qualitative Research*, 3rd edn. Thousand Oaks: Sage.

DePoy, E. & Gitlin, L.N. (2005) *Introduction to Research*, 3rd edn. St Louis: Mosby.

Grbich, C. (1999) *Qualitative Research in Health*. London: Sage.

Greenhalgh, T. (2006) *How to Read a Paper*, 3rd edn. Oxford: Blackwell Publishing.

Hammell, K.H., Carpenter, C. & Dyck, I. (2000) *Using Qualitative Research*. Edinburgh: Churchill Livingstone.

Holloway, I. (ed.) (2005) *Qualitative Research in Health Care*. Maidenhead: Open University Press.

Kielhofner, G. (1982) Qualitative research: part two, methodological approaches and relevance to occupational therapy. *Occupational Therapy Journal of Research* **2**, 150–170.

Krefting, L. (1991) Rigor in qualitative research: the assessment of trustworthiness. *American Journal of Occupational Therapy* **45**(3), 214–222.

Popay, J. & Williams, G. (1998) Qualitative research and evidence-based healthcare. *Journal of the Royal Society of Medicine* **91** (Suppl. 35), 32–37.

Strauss, A. & Corbin, J. (1998) *Basics of Qualitative Research: Techniques and Procedures for Developing Grounded Theory*, 2nd edn. California: Sage Publications.

Streubert, H.J. & Carpenter, D.R. (2006) *Qualitative Research in Nursing*, 4th edn. Philadelphia: JB Lippincott Co.

Yerxa, E.J. (1991) Seeking a relevant, ethical, and realistic way of knowing for occupational therapy. *American Journal of Occupational Therapy* **45**(3), 199–204.

6: Evidence from other sources

RCTs and systematic reviews will form the bulk of the types of research papers used by evidence-based occupational therapists when they attempt to explore the efficacy of their interventions, with additional supporting evidence drawn from qualitative research. However, these are not the only sources of potential evidence. As we discussed in Chapter 1, there is some debate about the nature of 'evidence' within evidence-based practice (EBP). This chapter aims to explore some of the other sources of evidence that might be used by the evidence-based occupational therapist to support and inform practice. The chapter will focus on three different sources of evidence: survey-based research; outcome methods; and the internet. Each source will be explored and its use within evidence-based occupational therapy (EBOT) outlined, with pointers to the questions to ask when critically appraising these different sources of evidence.

Survey-based research as sources of evidence

Survey-based research studies are designed to answer descriptive research questions, by producing a snapshot of a number of variables (or areas of interest) for a particular population (or group of people) at a particular time. Surveys can be used to describe a particular population in terms of its demographic details; an example of this type of survey would be a national census, which aims to provide a complete picture of the population of a country on a particular day. Other surveys will explore the ways people might vote or what people think or believe about a particular topic, such as patient satisfaction surveys. Variables within a survey may also be compared to see if there are any relationships or *correlations* between certain factors, such as social class and health or particular health behaviours and health outcomes.

Surveys have been a relatively popular research method within OT research, as the results of various database searches have shown (Table 6.1).

But what value does survey-based research have for EBOT? Surveys provide information about the demographics of a particular population or group of people; they can also give information about attitudes and beliefs relating to interventions or health behaviours, and they can give a picture of the prevalence of particular

Table 6.1 Searching for occupational therapy surveys.

Database	Search terms	Hits
CINAHL	occupational therapy AND surveys	873
AMED	occupational therapy AND surveys	315
MEDLINE	occupational therapy AND surveys	1003
Google	occupational therap* surveys	1470

Box 6.1 Surveys in OT

Brown *et al.* (2005) used a survey-based design to examine the nature of education about paediatric OT in the UK. In particular they explored the theoretical models, assessment tools and interventions that were taught, and compared what was taught with the literature and evidence base, to determine whether OT students in the UK were being taught the current best OT practice in the field of paediatric OT.

McKenna *et al.* (2005) used a survey design to explore the use of OTSeeker by Australian occupational therapists and their perceptions of the value and impact of OTSeeker on their knowledge and practice of both EBOT and also the impact on their clinical practice.

Eriksson *et al.* (2006) were interested in how people with an acquired brain injury adapted to their changed circumstances. They used a survey design to explore the occupational gaps for these individuals in terms of the differences between their actual everyday activities and what they wanted to be able to do. They were also interested in whether these gaps changed over time following the brain injury.

---

behaviours or illness (Box 6.1). This information can help the evidence-based occupational therapist in planning services and interventions. Surveys can also be used as ways of colleting expert opinion on particular topics as well as clients' opinions about the nature and quality of services. All of which may be used as evidence to guide the occupational therapist in decision-making about intervention choices.

Deane *et al.* (2001) attempted to develop a systematic review of the effectiveness of OT interventions for people with Parkinson's disease. However, they found that there was neither sufficient high-quality RCT evidence to support or challenge the effectiveness of OT interventions for people with Parkinson's disease, nor was there a consensus as to the best practice in OT when working with people with Parkinson's disease. As a result of these findings they carried out a survey of expert practitioners to discover what interventions occupational therapists were using and what they felt to be most effective when working with people with Parkinson's disease (Deane *et al.* 2003a, 2003b). Thus this survey-based information can be used by other occupational therapists to inform their choices about potential interventions for people with Parkinson's disease.

Data collection in survey-based research

Survey researchers use a variety of data collection methods. They include:

- questionnaires
- structured interviews
- Delphi questionnaires
- standardized questionnaires and measures

Questionnaires are by far the most commonly used data collection method. However, this is as much a limitation as a strength of this particular data collection method. As Oppenheim (1992) pointed out:

> A questionnaire is not just a list of questions or a form to be filled out. It is essentially a scientific instrument for measurement and for collection of particular kinds of data.

Unfortunately many researchers forget that a questionnaire is a rigorous scientific tool in their haste to put together a list of questions in order to find out what people think about a particular topic.

As we have already seen, qualitative research aims to explore people's beliefs and attitudes but is often seen as subjective. Questionnaires are thought of as the objective way of measuring behaviour, beliefs and attitudes (Oppenheim 1992). This is because, rather than ask people to express their thoughts in their own words, a questionnaire asks a series of questions about behaviour, beliefs, etc. and gives the respondent a range of options as to how to answer the question from a straightforward 'yes/no' through a range of alternatives to the commonly used Likert scale of 'strongly agree/agree/disagree/disagree strongly' (e.g. Yuker *et al.* 1960). Any questionnaire must be piloted to ensure that potential participants are able to understand and complete the questionnaire. Steps should also be taken to ensure that the questionnaire is valid and reliable.

For many aspects of health and illness behaviour, as well as in the field of attitude research, a wealth of standardized questionnaires and measures already exist (see Bowling 2001, 2004). These have the advantage that the validity and reliability of the questionnaire has already been assessed and established so that, as long as the measure is used correctly, the current study will also have some measure of validity and reliability (Box 6.2). A further benefit is that the findings of a number of studies utilizing the same measure can be compared.

Sampling in survey research

Having designed a data collection tool that is both valid and reliable, the rigour (and potentially the validity) of any survey-based research can still be flawed due to the nature of the population and the sampling process, which will govern whether the data can be generalized and how applicable the findings might be for the evidence-based occupational therapist.

Box 6.2 Data collection methods

Brown *et al.* (2005) used a self-administered questionnaire, which was distributed to participants by email. The questionnaire consisted of five sections, covering:

■ demographic information on the OT course;
■ information on the client diagnostic groups taught to students;
■ the paediatric theoretical models taught to students;
■ the assessments taught to students;
■ the interventions taught to students.

No further details of the questionnaire were given. The questionnaire was a modified version of a questionnaire that had been used in a number of previous studies of OT practitioners' views of paediatric OT practice. The questionnaire was piloted to ensure all relevant information had been included and that the format was clear and user-friendly. No further information on its validity and reliability was given.

McKenna *et al.* (2005) used a postal questionnaire to collect data in their study of the use of OTSeeker. The questionnaire was developed from a questionnaire used in two previous studies of clinicians' knowledge of EBP. The questionnaire consisted of three sections:

■ demographic information;
■ awareness and use of OTSeeker;
■ perceptions of the value and usefulness of OTSeeker.

No further information on the questionnaire was given. The questionnaire was piloted, but no information was given on the validity and reliability of the tool.

Eriksson *et al.* (2006) also used a postal questionnaire in their study of occupational gaps following brain injury. As well as demographic information, the questionnaire sought information about the participants' perceived impairments and their occupational behaviour and activities. The items within the questionnaire can be gleaned from the various result tables. The questionnaire does not appear to have been piloted and there is no information given about the validity and reliability of the tool.

Before we explore the various ways of sampling within survey-based research, we need to define two terms:

population is the term used to describe all of the members of the particular group of people the researcher is interested in – e.g. people with rheumatoid arthritis (RA), occupational therapists working with people with Parkinson's disease – however, it is rarely possible to collect data from everyone in the particular group of interest

sample is the term used to describe the people, and the process, selected to take part in the study

It is at the sampling stage that the study can become flawed, or biased, by over-representing particular subgroups within the sample (e.g. by age, gender, level of education). Coolican (1994) suggests that 85% of the studies within psychology have inadequate sampling methods. It might be interesting, and illuminating, to review the rigour of the sampling in the occupational therapy survey literature to see how rigorous the sampling has been.

Table 6.2 gives an overview of the varieties of sampling and the potential flaws that the evidence-based occupational therapist should be aware of when he or she is reviewing survey-based research.

But how many people constitutes a sufficient sample? The size of the sample will be influenced by a number of factors, including practical factors, such as the budget and resources available, as well as the size of the potential study population. Statisticians can calculate the optimal sample size for a given study population, but they will also caution against having too large, as well as too small, a sample. Large samples may add numbers but may also demonstrate the law of diminishing returns by acting to cloud rather than clarify the findings. It is important that the evidence-based occupational therapist looks carefully at the potential population for any study and then considers whether the sample best represents that population or might be too small to allow for representativeness (Box 6.3).

Equally important, however, is the response rate. Exactly how many of the potential participants actually completed the study and what did the researchers do to ensure a good response rate? Respondents feel more inclined to complete a questionnaire if it is clearly set out; if there are clear return instructions (including an SAE) or if they feel that they have a stake, or something to add, to the research. It is important that the evidence-based occupational therapist considers the non-responders, as well as the responders. There may be key differences between the people who responded to the study and those who chose not to respond, and these differences may impact on the validity of the findings of the study.

Appraising survey-based papers

The questions used to appraise survey-based studies are outlined in Table 6.3. These questions differ somewhat from the appraisal questions in the previous chapters although they are addressing essentially the same areas of validity, findings and applicability. The questions are inspired by a variety of sources, including Greenhalgh (2006), Gray (2001) and Crombie (1996).

Are the findings valid?

Has the research question been clearly stated?

As with any research it is important to know what the researchers' aims were and what research question they wanted their study to address. Without a clear research question the reader has no understanding of the nature of the research, or any way of assessing whether the findings have actually answered the original question.

Was a survey the appropriate design for the study?

The aim of any survey should be to address a descriptive research question, to describe what is happening at one point in time; to provide a snapshot of what

Table 6.2 Types of sampling within survey-based research.

Type of sample	Sampling process	Potential flaws
Random	Having identified the potential population, a random selection of people are invited to participate in the study. A computer is commonly used to make the random selection.	If it is possible to use a complete list of all the potential population, then this type of sampling will produce the least biased and most representative sample; however, perfect random sampling is rarely possible.
Stratified random	Before potential participants are selected they are divided into particular groups of interest to the researcher (e.g. age groups, gender, diagnostic groups). Random selection then takes place from each subgroup.	This method should produce a representative sample, but only if the chosen subgroupings are sufficiently varied. With small samples there will only be limited subgroups, which will limit the representation within the sample.
Quota	The researcher wants the sample to be representative of the proportions of key variables within the population (e.g. age, gender, etc.). However, the actual sampling is unlikely to be random. This method is commonly used by opinion poll researchers.	Whilst the sample may superficially appear to be representative of the population, there may be bias within each of the separate groups.
Snowball	More commonly used in qualitative research. One participant is asked to nominate other similar people who might be suitable to take part in the study.	May be biased. Method is very useful when trying to reach groups who are difficult to identify.
Convenience/opportunity	Participants are selected from a group who happen to be available. Often a pragmatic, rather than the ideal choice – e.g. asking all clients who happen to attend the department on a particular day.	This is the sampling method most likely to produce a biased sample as many people will not have the opportunity to be sampled.

Box 6.3 Sampling in OT survey-based research

Brown *et al.* (2005) studied the curriculum content for paediatric OT within UK-based OT pre-registration programmes. Their population was, therefore, relevant faculty members in all the 27 preregistration OT programmes in the UK. Given the small size of the study population, all 27 programmes were approached to take part in the study. The response rate was further enhanced by ensuring that the faculty member responsible for the paediatric content of the curriculum was contacted personally. Participants were informed of the nature of the study, and confidentiality and anonymity were assured. Reminders were sent 4 weeks after the initial email survey. Of the 27 potential respondents, 12 replied although only 10 provided usable data, which gave a response rate of 37%, which the authors considered to be adequate.

McKenna *et al.* (2005) used a postal questionnaire in their study of Australian occupational therapists' use of OTSeeker. Two random samples of Australian occupational therapists were used. The first sample sought to provide a national sample. OTAustralia is the national OT association and has approximately 4500 members. It is not clear whether all occupational therapists in Australia are members of the association. The potential population was stratified according to State/Territory and a random sample of 400 was selected. The sample size was dictated by resource availability. This resulted in what the researchers perceived to be a low response rate of 124 completed questionnaires, giving a response rate of 31%, even after two follow-up letters. It was therefore decided to sample occupational therapists working in two particular states (Queensland and New South Wales). Rather than target individual occupational therapists it was decided to target OT facilities. Approximately 10% (*n* = 95, giving a total of 487 occupational therapists) of the facilities on lists available to the researchers were targeted, and also received a follow-up telephone call. Completed questionnaires were returned by 89, representing a response rate of 27.3%. As there appeared to be no significant differences between the two samples the data were pooled, giving 213 completed responses to the study, from a potential OT population in the region of 4500.

Eriksson *et al.* (2006) used a postal questionnaire to explore the occupational gaps of people following acquired brain injury. The researchers drew their sample from the list of patients who had been treated for acquired brain injury at a particular hospital neurosurgical unit over the past 4 years. Inclusion criteria, as stated, were:

■ admission to intensive care for traumatic brain injury or subarachnoid haemorrhage;
■ aged between 20 and 65 years;
■ assessment during the acute phase by a rehabilitation physician.

A total of 217 questionnaires were sent out, although it is unclear whether questionnaires were sent to all eligible ex-patients. Follow-up reminders were sent out, and 187 completed questionnaires were returned, a very high response rate of 89%. Information was also provided about the 30 non-responders.

people are doing or of what they might think about a particular topic. Surveys cannot be used to assess whether one activity or intervention is more effective than another, although they can be used to assess what participants *think* might be most effective. Therefore if the study has goals beyond the descriptive, then the question might be more appropriately addressed by a different research design.

Table 6.3 Questions to ask when critically appraising a survey-based study.

Are the findings valid?
- Has the research question been clearly stated?
- Was a survey the appropriate design for the study?
- Was the data collection tool valid and reliable?
- Who was studied?
- How was the sample obtained?
- What was the response rate?
- How were the data analysed?

What are the findings?
- What are the main findings?
- Was the statistical significance assessed?
- Do the findings address the research question?
- What are the main conclusions?

How will these findings help me in my work with clients?
- Can the findings be generalized?
- Can the findings be applied to my practice?
- Can the study help me in my practice and my interactions with clients?

Was the data collection tool valid and reliable?

How did the researchers collect their data? Was the data collection tool valid; that is, did it measure what it was supposed to measure? Was the data collection tool reliable; that is, would it produce consistent results if the study were to be repeated? Two things help to ensure the validity and reliability of any data collection tool: a standardized questionnaire or measure, as long as the tool is used correctly; and a pilot trial of any data collection tool. What did the researchers do to ensure that their data collection tool was valid and reliable?

Who was studied?

The nature of the population and the sample for the study will influence how well the findings can be generalized. It is important that the researchers clearly set out the demographic parameters for the study (e.g. age, gender, diagnosis, profession). A clear description of the target population will also allow the reader to assess whether the sampling methods are appropriate.

How was the sample obtained?

As discussed above, sampling is vital to the validity of the findings of any survey research. Ideally everyone who might be considered to be eligible for the study should have an equal chance of being selected to participate. However, researchers often adopt a more convenience-based sampling process; they sample from the population they have at hand. How well was the sampling process described? Has the sample been drawn from a suitable range of potential participants or are key groups missing or under-represented?

What was the response rate?

The response rates of survey studies are notoriously low. A postal survey that elicits 30% of questionnaires returned is often regarded as a good response rate. What did the researcher do to ensure a high response rate? Were reminders sent out and non-responders contacted? Have the non-responders been identified and the impact of non-response discussed within the study? Does the non-response rate impact on the findings of the study?

How were the data analysed?

All surveys will require some level of statistical analysis, but exactly what did the researchers do? Did they use the correct statistical tests? What methods did they use to analyse any qualitative responses? Surveys tend to produce vast quantities of data, but look out for any evidence of 'data dredging'. Does it look as if the researchers have done all the possible tests their computer will allow in the hope that something comes out as a 'significant' result? Any analysis should be driven by a research question, not the other way round.

What are the findings?

What are the main findings?

How clearly have the findings been presented? Have any tables or graphs been clearly explained? Have key findings been linked to the research question and aims?

Was the statistical significance assessed?

Whilst many of the findings might relate to descriptive analysis, is there evidence of appropriate statistical analysis of the data? Have only the statistically significant findings been reported? What about any relevant non-significant findings?

Do the findings address the research question?

This links to the possibility of data dredging mentioned above. Look carefully at the findings, and review whether they do, in fact, address the research question.

What are the main conclusions?

What do the results actually mean? Do the conclusions drawn by the researchers link to the findings? How do the findings fit with the existing literature and knowledge within this topic? Have the researchers acknowledged the limitations of their study? Are the recommendations justified by the findings, or have the researchers made grand, global recommendations based on a very small local study?

How will these findings help me in my work with clients?

Can the findings be generalized?

This question draws on two areas; how well the sample matches the potential study population and how rigorous the study was. The latter question relates to the answers to the other appraisal questions, the former must be judged by looking at the non-response rate and at any other inherent biases within the sample.

Can the findings be applied to my practice?

Consider the population and the sample, how similar are they to your practice setting?

Can the study help me in my practice and my interactions with clients?

Are there useful messages that you can draw from this study that might help you to explore and develop your practice?

Finding the best outcome measures

As well as seeking research evidence to support their practice and interventions, evidence-based occupational therapists will draw on their own experiential evidence. This experiential evidence may be based on observations but should also be based on sound assessment and the evaluation of outcomes. But how is the evidence-based occupational therapist to identify which are the best and most rigorous assessment tools and outcome measures? This section will explore the nature of rigorous assessment and outcome measurement within OT and will offer some pointers to help the evidence-based occupational therapist in appraising the rigour and appropriateness of these tools and measures. It is, however, beyond the scope of this chapter to explore and debate the appropriateness of particular assessment tools and outcome measures in depth (see, e.g., Law *et al.* (2001) for an overview of outcome measures in OT; and Backman (2005) for a debate about the nature of outcomes within OT).

Assessment and outcome measurement in OT uses a variety of methods including structured (and unstructured) observation, interviews, activity- and performance-rating scales, and self-report. The tools may be standardized or non-standardized. Whilst an in-depth discussion of the value of standardized tools over non-standardized tools is outside the remit of this chapter, the emphasis within EBOT, and within this chapter, is on the use of standardized tools. Any assessment or outcome measure must be both valid and reliable. It must also be sufficiently sensitive to detect changes – this is known as responsiveness.

Before outlining how any assessment tool or outcome measure can be appraised, it is necessary to explore the concepts of validity, reliability and responsiveness. The terms validity and reliability will probably be familiar to the reader. However, it is important to make a distinction between the uses of these terms in the context of research design and the use of these terms here, in the context of assessment and measurement. In the research design context *reliability* refers to whether a study can be repeated and whether the same findings may occur. Having clear instructions and a clear research protocol should ensure this. *Validity*, in the research design context, is further divided into *internal validity* and *external validity*. The term internal validity refers to whether any differences within the study are genuinely the results of the intervention and not due to external factors, such as differences between therapists. External validity is about the extent to which findings can legitimately be applied to other people in other contexts. The terms validity and reliability are used somewhat differently in the context of measurement and assessment, as will be seen below.

Validity of assessment and outcome measures

The validity of an assessment or outcome measure refers to the extent to which the tool measures the thing that it has been designed to measure. For some things defining the phenomenon to be measured and whether the chosen measure is appropriate is relatively easy; for example, it is clear that bathroom scales are a valid measure of one's weight. However, other phenomena are more complex and so ensuring that a particular measure is valid is more difficult; for instance, stress, quality of life and Activities of Daily Living (ADL) are more complex and multi-faceted and so ensuring that a particular measure is actually measuring stress, quality of life or ADL is more complex, and would need to be assessed according to a number of the different forms of validity. The different forms of validity that can be assessed are:

■ face validity
■ content validity
■ criterion validity
■ predictive validity
■ construct validity

Face and content validity cannot be measured statistically. They refer to how well the measure appears to be assessing or measuring the whole of the phenomenon under assessment. Criterion validity, which is also known as concurrent validity, refers to how well the assessment tool of measure compares with the results of an existing valid measure of the same phenomenon or a 'gold standard' measure of the phenomenon. Statistical analysis would be a means of showing a correlation between the scores of the new tool and the existing tool. Predictive validity is only useful if the tool is being used to predict future outcomes (e.g. if a particular assessment score indicates the potential to be able to live independently in the community), and to assess this there must be a correlation either with that future outcome or with future scores on the gold standard assessment tool.

> **Box 6.4** Validity of an outcome measure
>
> Liepold and Mathiowetz (2005) developed the Self-Efficacy for Performing Energy Conservation Strategies Assessment (SEPECSA) for people with multiple sclerosis (MS). The measure was developed as part of a much larger study into the effectiveness of an energy conservation course, when previous measures were found to have little construct validity with self-efficacy theory and were not specific to MS. The SEPECSA consists of 14 items, based on the energy conservation strategies most likely to change as a result of the energy conservation course.
>
> The assessment measure appears to have face and content validity, as all 14 items on the scale specifically address levels of confidence in performing a range of energy conservation tasks.
>
> Construct validity was assessed by using the scale twice with the participants in the larger study, once before the energy conservation course and again at the end of the course. Each participant's scores were compared (using a paired t-test) to see if their self-efficacy had increased, as was predicted. The results were statistically significant. These results indicate that the scale does appear to have construct validity, as it provided a useful measure for a study of self-efficacy in energy conservation.

Many of the outcomes that occupational therapists are interested in can only be inferred from the subjective responses of the clients or others involved in their care; they cannot be measured directly. Unlike blood pressure or temperature, which can be objectively measured, quality of life or levels of fatigue rely on the client's subjective perceptions of a theoretical or hypothetical construct. The crucial factor for any assessment tool is that the construct that underpins the tool has coherence, or construct validity. Construct validity can be assessed in a number of ways. The measurement tool can be used within a research study where a particular phenomenon is being tested (Box 6.4). The ability of the various component parts of the tool to relate to each other can also be tested statistically, using factor analysis.

Reliability of assessment and outcome measures

The reliability of an assessment or measure demonstrates how likely it is that the measure will produce the same, or very similar, results on any number of occasions. The reliability of a measure is assessed through intra-rater testing (or test-retest), inter-rater testing and internal consistency assessment, and is supported by statistical analysis (Box 6.5). In intra-rater reliability, results from the same assessor should be consistent across time (i.e. assessing the same client(s) on different occasions). Inter-rater reliability refers to the consistency of results when two or more assessors test the same client(s). Internal consistency is assessed by comparing the results of individual questions, to ensure that participants are not contradicting themselves. A reliable assessment or measure is vital for the evidence-based occupational therapist. Without confidence in a reliable measure

Box 6.5 Reliability of an outcome measure

Liepold and Mathiowetz (2005) assessed the reliability of the SEPECSA by test-retest and internal consistency assessment.

Test-retest reliability was analysed using a variety of statistical tests, including correlation and *t*-tests. The results of these tests indicated that there were no significant differences and a high correlation on test-retest scores, indicating the reliability of the measure over time.

Internal consistency was analysed using Cronbach's α, which found a high level of internal consistency.

Overall, these results indicated that the SEPECSA is a reliable measure.

Box 6.6 Responsiveness of an outcome measure

The SEPECSA was used by Liepold and Mathiowetz (2005) to assess the impact of an energy conservation course. Significant improvements were noted in participants' scores, even though some participants had relatively high self-efficacy at the beginning of the energy conservation course. This indicated that the SEPECSA was a responsive measure and sensitive to changes in self-efficacy.

the evidence-based occupational therapist cannot be sure that any change in a client's function or occupational performance has occurred, and so cannot be sure whether the OT intervention has had any effect.

Whilst it is impossible for any OT measure to be completely reliable, statistical analysis during the development of any assessment or measure will give an indication of how reliable the tool should be. Three statistical tests are commonly used when assessing the intra- and inter-rater reliability of a measure, depending upon the type of data being collected. Percentage levels of agreement between assessors are used for binary scales (e.g. yes/no). Correlations and kappa analysis are used for more complex measures. Cronbach's α is used to measure internal consistency.

Responsiveness

Whilst it is vital for any assessment or outcome measure to be valid and reliable, it is also important that a tool can accurately record any changes in function or occupational performance. The ability of an assessment or measure to identify changes over time is known as *responsiveness* (Box 6.6). Often, as therapists, we notice important changes in our client's ability to function but when we reassess them these changes are not reflected in the assessment scoring system of our chosen measure. Thus it is important for the evidence-based occupational therapist to understand how sensitive any assessment or outcome measure might be and its ability to record changes over time.

Appraising assessments and outcome measures

The questions used to appraise assessment tools and outcome measures are outlined in Table 6.4. The questions are inspired by a variety of sources, including Jerosch-Herold (2005), Law *et al.* (2001) and Law (2002), and the writer's experiential knowledge.

Purpose of the assessment/outcome measure

What is the purpose of the assessment/outcome measure?

Has the purpose of the tool been clearly defined? Can it be used to predict future outcomes? Or is it purely an evaluative measure? Can it be used to aid diagnosis, as well as problem identification?

What is the definition of the construct of the tool/measure?

As we discussed above, many aspects of occupational performance and function are subjective and theoretical constructs. How clear is the construct being measured? How clear is the theoretical background to the construct and the measure? Does the measure have a sound OT focus and is it clearly linked to OT theory and models of practice?

Table 6.4 Questions to ask when critically appraising assessment tools and outcome measures.

Purpose of the assessment/outcome measure
■ What is the purpose of the assessment/outcome measure?
■ What is the definition of the construct of the tool/measure?
■ Who is the target for the tool/measure?

Practical information
■ Ease and feasibility of administration
■ Clarity of instructions
■ Scoring procedures
■ Assessor qualifications and training

Technical information and evaluation
■ Reliability
■ Validity
■ Responsiveness

External review and comments
■ What evidence of review is available?
■ What published literature is available to support or comment on the value of the tool/measure?

Summary of strengths and weaknesses
■ What are the key strengths and weaknesses of this tool/measure?
■ Will this tool/measure be of value with my clients and in my practice setting?

Who is the target for the tool/measure?

All assessments and outcome measures are designed with a particular group of people in mind, in terms of diagnostic group, ethnicity or age group. How similar are your clients to this group? Can the test be used in different cultural contexts? Although a tool/measure might be in English, it might have been designed with an American or Canadian context in mind; can this really translate to your particular practice context?

Practical information

Whilst appraising the practicalities of administering an assessment tool or outcome measure may seem odd, it is important to review the practicalities of administration. If a tool/measure is complex and time-consuming to administer a number of things can happen: either the tool/measure is rarely used or the tool/measure is misused, with parts of the tool/measure being used in isolation (a common mistake), which will impact on the validity and reliability of any standardized tool or measure. Appraising this information will also allow the evidence-based occupational therapist to assess the rigour of the standardization of the tool.

Ease and feasibility of administration

How feasible is the tool/measure to use? Do the instructions offer any guidance on modifications that might be permitted in order to facilitate the assessment of clients who are unable to fulfil the normal requirements of the tool/measure?

Clarity of instructions

Are the instructions sufficiently clear to ensure standardized administration of the tool/measure? Is the language appropriate for your client group? Will changing the language or instructions impact on the validity or reliability of the tool/measure?

Scoring procedures

Are the scoring procedures clearly described? Is the scoring easy to interpret? Is the scoring sufficiently sensitive to indicate change? Do the instructions also discuss the interpretation and possible predictive value of the tool/measure?

Assessor qualifications and training

Some tools/measures require additional qualifications or attendance at courses (e.g. AMPS). What are the qualifications required for this tool/measure? Does it need a qualified occupational therapist? What are the implications of these training requirements? Can the tool/measure be self-administered?

Technical information and evaluation

Reliability

What measures have been taken to ensure test-retest reliability, internal consistency and inter-rater reliability? What statistical analysis of reliability has been presented and how strong are the correlations between scores?

Validity

Does the tool/measure have face validity? What measures have been used to ensure content and construct validity? Has the validity of the tool/measure been adequately demonstrated?

Responsiveness

What evidence is presented for the sensitivity and responsiveness of the tool? Is there evidence that it can accurately record small changes in function or occupational performance over time and across a range of client abilities?

External review and comments

What evidence of review is available?

Has the tool been subjected to any external review? Has the tool been used in any research contexts, where it has been found to be of value?

What published literature is available to support or comment on the value of the tool/measure?

How widespread is the use of this measure in the OT (or other) literature? Has the tool been utilized in a variety of settings or in a variety of contexts? What evidence is there of published literature to support the value of this tool?

Summary of strengths and weaknesses

What are the key strengths and weaknesses of this tool/measure?

By this stage you should be able to draw up a list of the potential strengths and limitations of this tool/measure. This information will help you to judge whether the tool/measure has utility and potential value for your practice setting.

Will this tool/measure be of value with my clients and in my practice setting?

Having completed your review of the assessment tool/outcome measure, what conclusions can you draw about its potential value within your own practice setting? Is it appropriate for your client group? Is it sufficiently robust? How well will the tool/measure fit with the practice of other professionals in your practice setting?

Using the internet as a source of evidence

The internet is a very powerful and accessible tool, providing us with access to huge amounts of information from around the world. Many millions of people access information via the internet on a daily basis, and it is estimated that at least half of these are trying to gain information about health, illness and treatment options (Risk & Petersen 2002; Powell *et al.* 2003). The internet is a resource that is available not only to the evidence-based occupational therapist but also to her or his clients and their carers. But how can the occupational therapist sift through, or help their clients to sift through, all the available information to find useful and sound information?

Eysenbach and Köhler (2002) and Peterson *et al.* (2003) explored the use of internet-based health information and found that many people do not remember where they retrieved information or check the identity or origin of the information, and thus have no idea whether the information is reputable or of high quality. The internet is predominantly unregulated and unaccountable and the information available is of highly variable quality. It is vital that evidence-based occupational therapists have the skills critically to appraise the quality of any internet-based information and have a variety of high-quality sources at their disposal, or at least bookmarked on their 'favourites' list. Many of these potential resources are discussed in Chapter 10 (Useful resources). However, before discussing what questions to use when appraising internet-based evidence, a number of web-based resources that might be of particular value to the evidence-based occupational therapist will be discussed.

OTseeker (www.otseeker.com)

OTseeker, a database modelled on PEDro (the Physiotherapy Evidence Database; www.pedro.fhs.usyd.edu.au), was launched in March 2003 (McClusky *et al.* 2006). OTseeker is a database of RCTs and systematic reviews of relevance to occupational therapists. The database is freely available. All RCTs on the database have been quality assessed by two trained assessors, using the PEDro rating scale (Maher *et al.* 2003). Searches of the database are listed according to methodological quality, with systematic reviews appearing first, followed by the highest quality RCTs. All entries include full citation information and most contain the article's abstract and, where possible, links to the full text of the article. This database is an extremely valuable web-based resource for the evidence-based occupational therapist.

Evidence Based Occupational Therapy portal (www.otevidence.info)

The Evidence Based Occupational Therapy portal is a much more recent resource, having been launched in July 2006 at the 14th World Federation of Occupational Therapists (WFOT) Congress. The portal has been designed by an international collaboration of occupational therapists to provide knowledge, resources and strategies to assist occupational therapists in finding out about and using evidence within OT practice. The portal includes opportunities for web-based discussions as well as educational and teaching resources for EBP and EBOT, and links to databases and other internet EBP resources. One of the most important features of the portal is in providing free full-text access to a number of articles on EBP and EBOT that would otherwise only be available via subscription. The portal is still in its infancy, but it should prove to be another valuable internet resource for the evidence-based occupational therapist.

Appraising internet-based evidence

The questions used to appraise assessment tools and outcome measures are outlined in Table 6.5. The questions are inspired by a variety of sources, including Eysenbach and Köhler (2002), Risk (2002) and Kiley (2003).[1]

Table 6.5 Questions to ask when critically appraising internet-based information.

Source of the information
■ What is the source and origin of the information?
■ Who is the author?
■ Is there evidence of funding or sponsorship?
■ Is there evidence of a quality seal or other quality mechanisms?
■ Is there an opportunity for feedback or to contact the author?

Content of the website
■ What is the scope and aims of the information?
■ Who is the intended audience?
■ How accurate is the information?
■ Is the information up to date?
■ How relevant is the content to your needs?
■ Is the content presented at an appropriate level for the intended audience?
■ Is there evidence of bias?

Design and layout of the website
■ Is the information clearly presented?
■ Are the design and layout accessible?
■ Are navigation and searching of the site clear?
■ Are any external links appropriate and active?

Applicability of the information
■ Does this site provide information that will be of value to my practice?

[1] Other sources of appraisal and guidance when using internet-based evidence can be found at: DISCERN (www.discern.org.uk) – a brief series of questions to help users appraise information on treatment choices.

Source of the information

What is the source and origin of the information?

Websites are produced by a wide variety of organizations and individuals, ranging from companies trying to sell their products, through universities and researchers trying to disseminate information, to individuals with a particular illness who want to share their particular perspective. As well as being able to identify the author of the information (see next question) it is useful and illuminating to be able to extract as much information as possible from the uniform resource locator (URL, or web address). The affix '.com' or '.co' usually indicates a commercial organization; the affix '.ac' or '.edu' indicates a university or academic institution; '.org' is usually a non-profit-making or charitable organization; '.gov' indicates a government department. Apart from websites hosted in the USA, all URLs finish with the country of origin; for example '.uk' and '.au'. Look carefully at the URL – what can you glean from it about the source of the information?

Who is the author?

Is the author clearly identified? What are the author's credentials? Is the author appropriately qualified and with suitable and relevant knowledge and experience to provide this information?

Is there evidence of funding or sponsorship?

Is there any evidence of who might be funding the site? Some sites will be sponsored by third parties. If there is evidence of sponsorship, often identifiable by a logo, who is the sponsor? Is there likely to be a potential for bias because of the nature of the sponsorship? Is there evidence of advertising or links to advertisement on the site, which might indicate external involvement in the content or potential conflicts of interest?

Is there evidence of a quality seal or other quality mechanisms?

Organizations such as the Health on the Net Foundation (www.hon.ch) provide guidelines and codes of conduct for promoting high standards on websites, and sites that meet their standards can display the appropriate logo, demonstrating a level of confidence in the quality of information (Wilson 2002).

Is there an opportunity for feedback or to contact the author?

Being able to contact the author allows you to respond to the information, to comment on the usefulness of the site, to engage in discussion with the author or to identify any errors.

Content of the website

What are the scope and aims of the information?

Does the site state any aims, or have a mission statement? Is its scope clearly identified? Do the 'help' section or FAQs give any information about the scope or aims of the site?

Who is the intended audience?

Is it clear who the information is aimed at? Is the information for the general public or more specifically aimed at healthcare professionals?

Is the content presented at an appropriate level for the intended audience?

As well as being accurate, information should be presented at a level that is appropriate for the audience. If it is aimed at the general public then it should be worded appropriately and easy to understand, without excessive use of jargon or terminology.

How relevant is the content to your needs?

Information about health and social care practice does not always translate well into different settings or different countries. How well can the information be applied to your context? The internet gives us access to an enormous amount of information, but this can mean we get side-tracked by interesting but irrelevant information. Does the information address your original evidence-based question?

How accurate is the information?

Based on your knowledge of this topic, how accurate is the information presented on the website? Have all relevant areas been covered? Comments such as 'studies have shown' should be supported by references or links to relevant supporting material. Are supporting references and links accurate and appropriate?

Is the information up to date?

Information, particularly health-related information, can become out of date very quickly. When was the site last updated? Is there evidence that the information is reviewed regularly? If the site is not updated regularly, this could indicate that information may be past its use-by date, or has been superseded by new information.

Is there evidence of bias?

Is the information presented in a balanced and neutral manner? Are all sides of the story given equal weight? Are the authors trying to persuade you in any way?

Does the site claim to be the only reliable source of information? Does the site denigrate any other sites? If the answer to these last two questions is 'yes' treat the information contained on this site with great caution (UK Health Centre 2002).

Design and layout of the website

Is the information clearly presented?

Whilst the layout and design of a site may not be the best criteria for judging the quality of the information, they will have an impact on whether the site is used and the information is read. Is information presented clearly? Is there an index to what the site contains? Is the presentation of information logical? Is the information well written and easy to understand?

Are the design and layout accessible?

Guidelines exist to ensure that information on the web is accessible to everyone, which means ensuring that the information is easily accessible to people with disabilities. How easy is the site to use for someone with a disability?

Are navigation and searching of the site clear?

How easy is it to find your way around the various sections of the site? A well-organized site not only makes it easier to find relevant information but also indicates that appreciable work has gone into the development of the site. Is it possible to search the site for particular information? How well does this search facility work?

Are any external links appropriate and active?

If the site includes links to other internet sites, are these links still active? Are there any 'dead' (or inactive) links? Dead links might imply that the site is not updated regularly and so might indicate that any information is also out of date. Are the links of good quality? Links to poor-quality sites might reflect on the credibility of this site.

Applicability of the information

Does this site provide information that will be of value to my practice?

Having completed your review of the website and its information, what conclusions can you draw about its potential value within your own practice setting? Is it appropriate for your client group?

▪ ▪

Activities

- Identify a survey-based study of relevance to your area of practice/interest.
- Using the appraisal questions above, work with a colleague to appraise the article and to assess its value as evidence.
- List all of the outcome measures and assessment tools used within your department/service.
- Using the strategy outlined above, work with a colleague to appraise each tool and to assess its value and appropriateness.
- Use Google to search for evidence to support your practice.
- Using the questions outlined above, work with a colleague to appraise any website you find and to assess its value as a source of evidence.
- Use OTseeker to look for research papers that are of relevance to your practice, and discuss the value of OTseeker as a potential EBOT resource with your colleagues.

▪ ▪

Further reading

The following references will allow the reader to explore issues pertinent to the understanding and appraisal of different sources of evidence in more depth.

Backman, C. (2005) Outcomes and outcome measures: measuring what matters is in the eye of the beholder. *Canadian Journal of Occupational Therapy* **72**(5), 259–264.

Boynton, P.M. (2004) A hands on guide to questionnaire research, part two: administering, analysing, and reporting your questionnaire. *British Medical Journal* **328**, 1372–1375.

Boynton, P.M. & Greenhalgh, T. (2004) A hands on guide to questionnaire research, part one: selecting, designing, and developing your questionnaire. *British Medical Journal* **328**, 1312–1315.

Boynton, P.M., Wood, G.W. & Greenhalgh, T. (2004) A hands on guide to questionnaire research, part three: reaching beyond the white middle classes. *British Medical Journal* **328**, 1433–1436.

Kiley, R. (2003) *Medical Information on the Internet*. Edinburgh: Churchill Livingstone.

Law, M., Baum, C. & Dunn, W. (2001) *Measuring Occupational Performance*. Thorofare, NJ: Slack Incorporated.

Oppenheim, A.N. (1992) *Questionnaire Design, Interviewing and Attitude Measurement*. Thousand Oaks: Sage.

7: Making evidence-based practice work

The importance of clinical effectiveness and evidence-based practice is emphasized in UK government policy (NHS Executive 1996; Walshe 1998). The creation of a National Institute for Health and Clinical Excellence (NICE), with its emphasis on evaluating the effectiveness of healthcare interventions, both in terms of cost and clinical effectiveness, supports this policy (Department of Health 1997). In 2004, the World Federation of Occupational Therapists established an International Advisor Group on Evidence-based Practice (Piergrossi 2004). However, as Newell (1997) states, much of the impetus for clinical effectiveness and evidence-based practice is focused at institutional levels. Others (e.g. Bury 1998; Keep 1998; Needham & Oliver 1998) have written about the management aspects of making evidence-based healthcare work. The focus of this book has been much more practical. This chapter will, therefore, focus on practical ways in which occupational therapists can become involved in evidence-based practice, by using reflection, supervision and mentoring, and through journal clubs and evidence-based audit of existing practice. However, the perceived barriers to evidence-based practice must be acknowledged and the chapter will conclude by looking at ways of identifying and overcoming the barriers to evidence-based occupational therapy (EBOT) and using theories of research utilization and change management to establish an evidence-based culture for OT practice.

Using evidence-based practice in the practice/intervention setting

The requirement to use the best available research evidence when making intervention decisions is now enshrined within the standards for professional practice in OT set by professional and statutory bodies (e.g. College of Occupational Therapists 2003, 2005; Health Professions Council 2003) and for OT professional education internationally (Hocking & Ness 2002). All occupational therapists have an ethical responsibility to be:

> personally responsible for actively maintaining and developing their personal development and professional competence
>
> (College of Occupational Therapists 2005, para. 5.4)

and to

> be accountable for the quality of their work and base this on current guidance, research, reasoning and best available evidence
>> (College of Occupational Therapists 2005, para. 5.4.3)

This national imperative is further reinforced internationally by the World Federation of Occupational Therapists (WFOT) Code of Ethics, which states:

> Occupational therapists participate in professional development through life-long learning and apply their acquired knowledge and skills in their professional work which is based on the best available evidence
>> (World Federation of Occupational Therapists 2004)

This places the onus on all practitioners to become evidence-based occupational therapists. However, as we have seen, the potential sources of research evidence pertinent to OT are large. The average occupational therapist has little hope of managing to read *everything* pertinent to her or his field of practice.

Using reflection, supervision and mentoring to become an evidence-based occupational therapist

Many therapists wonder how to become involved in evidence-based practice without realizing that they are already working within an evidence-based perspective. The processes of reflection, supervision and discussion with a mentor are all opportunities to review one's practice from an evidence-based perspective. Evidence-based practice, as we have seen, is not about *doing* research but about *using* research very explicitly to underpin the intervention decisions we make on a daily basis as practitioners.

As occupational therapists we are encouraged to be reflective practitioners, to look critically at what we do. The process of reflection involves describing an event and then looking at the decision-making and reasoning process, which underpins the actions taken within that event. The event concerned can be any interaction with a client. These reflections can form the basis of supervision or mentoring discussions.

To make the reflective process evidence-based it is necessary to address the following questions:

- Is there any evidence to underpin the intervention decisions I made in this situation?
- Have I searched for the evidence to underpin this intervention?
- Am I using evidence to underpin the decisions I made in this situation?
- Have I critically appraised this evidence?
- Are there any professional, national or local standards and guidelines that are relevant to this intervention and situation?
- Have I critically appraised this information?
- Am I involving the client in the decisions about intervention?

■ Am I informing the client of the evidence base for these interventions?
■ Am I regularly updating my knowledge?
■ Am I sharing and disseminating the evidence I have gathered?

Reflective and evidence-based practice should not be threatening. By thinking through and articulating the reasoning processes we use, unconsciously, every day we can strengthen, rather than weaken, our practice. Outdated and redundant interventions can be stopped and effective interventions can be reinforced.

Student occupational therapists on fieldwork placements can be a useful aid to the evidence-based occupational therapist. Students are encouraged to be reflective and they are encouraged to question and explore the clinical reasoning processes they are using. They also have search and research skills and access to their university libraries. As part of their reflections on the interventions they are involved with students should be encouraged to search for and present the evidence to underpin the interventions.

Journal clubs

One way of ensuring focused reading, and developing an evidence-based climate, is to establish a *journal club*. Journal clubs are groups of people (from three to ten members) who meet regularly (every one or two months) to review and discuss one or more articles of relevance to their practice. Journal clubs can provide useful opportunities to practise the critical appraisal skills discussed in the previous chapters. Membership of, and commitment to, a journal club could provide useful evidence of continuing professional development for an individual's professional portfolio and performance review.

Journal clubs have been a part of medical practice for many years (Linzer 1987). These journal clubs often consisted of one person presenting a critical review of an article to her or his colleagues. However, as Sackett *et al.* (1997) point out, this type of journal club is becoming extinct. A much more successful, and useful, format for journal clubs, advocated by Sackett *et al.* (1997) and Linzer *et al.* (1988), is a journal club based on a critical appraisal format. Here a group of colleagues meet together to share a discussion and appraisal of one or more papers, probably using an appraisal checklist (see previous chapters) as a way of structuring the discussion.

Journal clubs, using an appraisal format, not only provide a forum for practising appraisal skills, but can also provide an opportunity to review and reflect upon current practice. The outcome of a journal club discussion may be to implement changes to current interventions or practice. The journal club can provide a valuable opportunity for colleagues to explore issues, share ideas, consider differing perspectives and participate in the shaping and developing of departmental practice and policy. Box 7.1 gives an overview and format for establishing a journal club.

Box 7.1 Establishing a journal club

Planning

For a journal club to run well, it needs to be planned and organized; members should be committed to the success of the group.

- Leadership – the journal club needs an overall convenor who will lead and plan meetings, although each meeting can be led by different members of the group.
- Membership – the size of the group should be from three to ten people who are committed to the idea of the journal club.
- Establish regular meetings – set a timetable and plan meetings in advance; decide on a regular time and day for the meetings.
- Find a location – identify a suitable, informal location where the club can meet, with minimal interruptions. Meetings could be combined with lunch.
- Decide on the themes to be discussed – this might take place at the first meeting of the group. Decide on clear evidence-based questions with clearly identified problems, interventions and outcomes. Decide who will be responsible for organizing and running each session.
- Liaise with the librarian – having established the themes/evidence-based questions, each session leader will need to find relevant articles for the group to discuss. Work with your librarians to find the articles.
- Distribute/photocopy articles – make sure that all members of the group have access to copies of the articles for discussion at least a week before the meeting.

The meeting

- Use an appraisal checklist (see previous chapters).
- Set clear time limits – spend the majority of the session discussing the chosen article(s), but allow time at the end of the session to discuss the implications for your department and to make an action plan if changes are to be made.
- Avoid 'critical appraisal nihilism' (Sackett *et al.* 1997, p. 193) – all research has flaws, but most research can be useful.
- Don't get 'tied up' on the numbers – focus on the key outcomes rather than whether a *t*-test really was the best analysis.
- Make sure that everyone has a chance to join in.
- Establish an 'open' climate, where any contribution is accepted and valued.
- Have fun and enjoy the discussions.

Follow-up

- Make sure that any action plans, reflections or ideas for change are referred to the appropriate people.
- Keep notes of the topics discussed and the outcomes.

Journal clubs can be uniprofessional or multidisciplinary. Which is the most appropriate will depend on your setting. Each meeting can consider a single article or a number of articles. Single articles can be useful to start with, as everyone develops their appraisal skills. However, although looking at a number of papers may take longer, it will give a broader and more interesting perspective on any given topic or evidence-based question.

Journal clubs do require time and an element of commitment. Given the current climate of clinical effectiveness and continuing professional development, managers should encourage and facilitate the establishment of journal clubs. Searching for relevant articles may feel like an onerous responsibility, but if searching and session leadership are divided among the group members it should not prove too difficult and time consuming a task.

■ ■

Activity

Establish a journal club:

- ■ Collect together a group of like-minded colleagues.
- ■ Establish a time for regular meetings.
- ■ Decide on a number of evidence-based questions and allocate the planning of each session.
- ■ Meet as a journal club.

■ ■

Evidence-based audit

Another approach that all occupational therapists can use to incorporate evidence into their practice is through evidence-based audit. Audit has been part of the UK's National Health Service (NHS) policy for a number of years (Department of Health 1991), and can be defined as:

> The systematic critical appraisal of the quality of clinical care including the procedures for diagnosis, treatment and care, the associated use of resources and the resulting outcome and quality of life for the patient.
>
> (NHS Management Executive 1994)

The systematic process of audit has involved establishing standards and protocols for intervention and care and using these standards and protocols to review the quality of care received by clients. The focus of audit has been on enhancing and improving the *quality* of health and social care. Standards and protocols of care have been established but they have rarely been based on evidence. However, the current climate of health and social care focuses on *clinical effectiveness* (NHS Executive 1996). This has placed the emphasis on the synthesis of audit and evidence-based practice, resulting in the development of the process of *evidence-based audit*. Table 7.1 summarizes the similarities and differences between audit and evidence-based audit.

The focus of audit has been to set standards and guidelines based on local knowledge and expertise. The focus of evidence-based audit is to add research evidence to the expertise and experience of local practitioners. The process of developing and auditing clinical (or intervention) guidelines will be discussed in the next section. It is not the function of this book to give a step-by-step account of the evidence-based audit process. Rather, the aim of this book is to highlight how the reader can become an evidence-based occupational therapist and to highlight the resources available to develop his or her skills. Numerous books and articles have been published on the process of audit and evidence-based audit, including Buttery (1996), Kogan *et al.* (1995), Malby (1995) and Arnold *et al.* (1995). All NHS Trusts should have clinical effectiveness and/or clinical audit departments that will be delighted to help in the development of evidence-based audit of local OT services. Evidence-based audit should not be a solitary task, although it can be used as a process for reflecting upon and reviewing your own practice. A much better approach to evidence-based audit is for a group of colleagues, within one intervention setting, to work together to review, reflect upon and audit their interventions and practice. The process of evidence-based audit might lead to the development of local guidelines for practice and interventions.

Activity

- Meet with a number of colleagues to reflect on practice and to develop topics for evidence-based audit.
- Identify and locate the clinical effectiveness/audit personnel within your NHS Trust or service setting.
- Discuss the topics for evidence-based audit with the clinical effectiveness/audit personnel.
- Establish an audit strategy for your setting.

Table 7.1 Comparison of audit and evidence-based audit.

Audit	Evidence-based audit
Identify clinical audit topic	Identify clinical audit topic
	Find relevant research evidence and expert information
	Critically appraise the evidence
Agree standards, protocols and guidelines	Agree evidence-based standards, protocols and guidelines
Implement standards, protocols, guidelines	Implement evidence-based standards, protocols, guidelines
Assess compliance with standards, protocols and guidelines	Assess compliance with evidence-based standards, protocols and guidelines
Review standards, protocols and guidelines	Review evidence-based standards, protocols and guidelines (this will involve finding and appraising any new evidence)
Agree changes (if required)	Agree changes (if required)
Implement reviewed and refined standards, protocols and guidelines	Implement reviewed and refined standards, protocols and guidelines

A model for an evidence-based OT process

Whilst supervision, reflection and journal clubs can help the evidence-based occupational therapist to develop the skills of evidence-based practice, they do not always ensure that the practice and interventions of OT are truly evidence-based. For this we need an evidence-based approach to the OT process. Rappolt (2003) has proposed an, as yet untested, model of a client-centred evidence-based OT process, which acknowledges the need to integrate the three strands of evidence (from the client, from research and from professional experience) into the OT process. The model is presented in Fig. 7.1.

The potential value of this model is that it clearly identifies not only a collaborative approach to evidence-based OT between the therapist and the client, it also identifies where research expertise and skills (as in stage 2) and professional experiential knowledge (as in stage 3) are of potential value in the decision-making process. It is hoped that this model might provide a usable framework for the development of truly evidence-based OT practice.

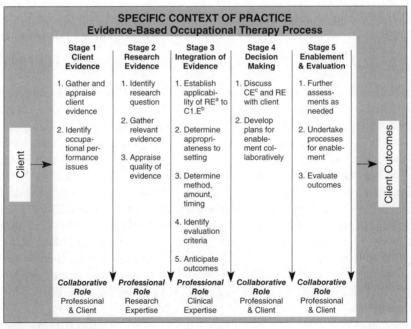

^a RE = Research evidence
^b C1.E = Client evidence
^c CE = Clinical expertise

Figure 7.1 Rappolt's (2003) model for a client-centred evidence-based OT process. Reproduced with permission from the American Occupational Therapy Association.

Barriers to evidence-based practice

A growing body of evidence exists suggesting that occupational therapists – and other PAMS (professions allied to medicine) colleagues – are not confident evidence-based practitioners (Turner & Whitefield 1996, 1997; Brown 1998; Wiles & Barnard 1998; Dubouloz *et al.* 1999; Upton 1999a, 1999b; Pollock *et al.* 2000; Curtin & Jaramazovic 2001; Cameron *et al.* 2005; Welch & Dawson 2006) and that a number of factors must be considered when attempting to implement evidence-based practice (EBP) (Pain *et al.* 2004; Rycroft-Malone *et al.* 2004; Thurston & King 2004). Upton (1999a) and Pollock *et al.* (2000) found that occupational therapists held very positive attitudes towards the value of EBP. However, they rated their EBP knowledge and skills as low, especially in terms of the technical skills of EBP. Upton (1999a) defined the technical skills of EBP as information technology (IT) skills, literature-searching skills and research skills. Turner and Whitefield (1996, 1997), Wiles and Barnard (1998) and Welch and Dawson (2006) all found that therapists, whilst accepting the need for evidence-based approaches to practice, tended to rely on personal experience, practice-related courses and professional craft knowledge when selecting interventions. Wiles and Barnard (1998) found that physiotherapists perceived potential conflicts between:

■ EBP and existing experiential knowledge;
■ EBP and patient-orientated practice;
■ EBP practice and the independent and autonomous status of practitioners.

Sumsion (1997) has also highlighted the potential conflict between EBP and client-centred philosophies of practice.

The need for occupational therapists to embrace EBP has also been recognized and encouraged with special issues of both the *British Journal of Occupational Therapy* (College of Occupational Therapists 1997) and the *Canadian Journal of Occupational Therapy* (Canadian Association of Occupational Therapists 1998, 2003) dedicated to EBP, conferences on EBP in mental health (British Journal of Therapy and Rehabilitation 1996), the regular 'Evidence-based Practice Forum' in the *American Journal of Occupational Therapy*, and the establishing of the critically appraised papers (CAPs) section in the *Australian Occupational Therapy Journal*. However, a number of authors (e.g. Taylor 1997; Clemence 1998; Wilson-Barnett 1998) have highlighted the potential conflict between the qualitative research methodologies favoured by nursing and OT and the high status given to randomized controlled trials (RCTs) in EBP. This should present less of a problem in the future with the growing acceptance of qualitative research within EBP (Popay & Williams 1998).

Whilst EBP and evidence of clinical effectiveness are the driving forces in current health and social care, there are a number of barriers to the utilization of EBP by OTs. These barriers are summarized in Table 7.2.

Upton's (1999b) research identified, in descending order of importance, the following factors, which would increase the use of evidence-based approaches to practice:

Table 7.2 Barriers to evidence-based practice (EBP).

Access to, and availability of, information
Limited time
Lack of EBP skills
Lack of confidence in the value of the evidence that is available
Lack of support from management and colleagues
Conflict with the client-centred philosophy of OT

- more time;
- better dissemination;
- greater library resources;
- money;
- greater availability of IT;
- greater commitment from management;
- better access to the internet.

The various barriers, highlighted in Table 7.2, can be overcome, although commitment to change is also a vital ingredient of the process of developing an EBOT culture.

Access to, and availability of, information

Access to the relevant information can be seen in terms of having access to suitable library resources and also being able to find the relevant information in the vast array of journals available to the evidence-based occupational therapist. Access to this range of information may become easier with the increased use of electronic rather than paper-based journals, allowing evidence-based occupational therapists to access relevant material from the comfort of their own computer. However, access may also be limited because of lack of dissemination of research findings. Research evidence may only be available in the 'grey' (or unpublished) literature. Research findings may be presented at conferences but never make it into print. More and more conferences are now using the internet as a means of giving access to conference proceedings, which will help the evidence-based occupational therapist to begin to access some of the grey literature.

Limited time

Time, for most occupational therapists, is often a scarce commodity. However, time for EBP activity can be acknowledged, possibly through the performance review system, and the need for all practitioners to demonstrate ongoing learning and continuing professional development (CPD) activity.

Lack of EBP skills

The key EBP skills that appear to be needed are:

- IT skills;
- literature searching skills;
- critical appraisal skills.

The Critical Appraisal Skills Programme (CASP) workshops (see Chapter 10) can be used to address both searching and appraisal skills development. These skills can then be cascaded throughout a department.

A useful strategy would be to audit the evidence-based skills within the department; not only in terms of actual skill but also in terms of the confidence each team member has in those skills. This information can then be used to formulate a strategy to encourage the development of skills and confidence in skills throughout the department.

Confidence in the value of the evidence that is available

There is a growing body of evidence (e.g. Wiles & Barnard 1998; Upton 1999b; Welch & Dawson 2006) that therapists are less willing to act on research evidence than they are to act on other forms of evidence to review or change their practice. Upton (1999b) found, in descending order of willingness to act, that therapists would act on information from the following sources:

- own practice and experience;
- colleagues from the same profession;
- line manager;
- journal articles;
- clinical effectiveness facilitator;
- colleagues from different professions;
- the internet.

when reviewing or changing their practice. From this evidence there would appear to be a mismatch between the accepted hierarchy of evidence for EBP and the value therapists place on various sources of evidence.

Perhaps one of the biggest challenges to the development of EBOT is this reliance upon experiential knowledge. However, the definition of EBOT cited earlier emphasizes the use of three strands of evidence when making intervention decisions. The evidence-based occupational therapist should draw on her or his own experiential evidence, on evidence and information from the client and on a critical review of the research evidence. As we have seen, research evidence can encompass everything from systematic reviews to single qualitative studies, and experiential evidence can be strengthened by the use of rigorous assessment tools and outcome measures. The skill is to synthesize all of this evidence and to make sure that all three strands are utilized rather than to concentrate on experiential evidence alone.

Support from management and colleagues

Establishment of an evidence-based culture must come from both managers and practitioners. Journal clubs (see above) can be useful ways of beginning to develop an evidence-based culture within a department. The objectives set as part of the development and appraisal process can be used to underpin the development of an evidence-based culture, by making the goals of finding, appraising and using evidence explicit, thus ensuring that time should be allocated to evidence-based activity.

Conflict with the client-centred philosophy of OT

If EBP is seen, as Sackett *et al.* (1997) propose, as the judicious use of current best evidence, then there is no conflict between an evidence-based and a client-centred philosophy of practice. Upton (1999a, 1999b) identifies 'involving patients fully in their care' as a key component of EBP. This aspect of EBP was the component most frequently used by the therapists in Upton's research. Discussing the effectiveness of proposed interventions with any client can only enhance the client-centred philosophy of any occupational therapist's practice.

Brown (1998) proposes the following strategies as useful for practitioners wanting to become evidence-based occupational therapists:

■ Adopt a 'spirit of enquiry';
■ Read widely and critically;
■ Attend professional conferences;
■ Become involved in a journal club;
■ Collaborate with a researcher;
■ Develop strategic alliances.

For the manager wishing to develop an evidence-based culture, the following strategies might be useful:

■ Foster a climate of intellectual curiosity;
■ Offer emotional and moral support;
■ Offer resources and financial support;
■ Reward evidence-based initiatives and efforts;
■ Be a role model and a mentor.

The most common barrier to becoming an evidence-based occupational therapist is an ambivalence about the meaning of 'evidence' (Taylor 2003) and a tendency to rely on experiential rather than research evidence (Turner & Whitefield 1997, 1999; Pringle 1999). Sackett *et al.* (1996, 1997) recognized that EBP must include a synthesis of both research and experiential knowledge. The challenge is to find a way of incorporating both experiential and research evidence within any model of research utilization and to use change management theories to facilitate the development of an evidence-based culture within the work setting.

Models of research utilization

A number of models of research utilization exist. A selection of these models will be outlined and discussed to evaluate their usefulness for the change to EBOT. The final model to be discussed is one that is specific to OT.

Research utilization has a number of definitions, but essentially it is a process whereby research findings are critiqued, implemented into practice and their implementation evaluated. The impact of research utilization is either specific to one client or area of practice or generalized in order to increase understanding and promote enlightenment throughout professional practice (Brown & Rodger 1999). All of which sounds very similar to the process of EBP. However, there are significant differences between EBP and research utilization. The models of research utilization focus on the use of research within practice. Within EBP the use of research is just one component of the evidence that evidence-based occupational therapists might utilize in their intervention decisions and clinical reasoning.

Knott and Wildavsky (1980) were probably the first to develop a model for research (or knowledge) utilization into practice. They proposed a series of stages to demonstrate the thinking processes that might be involved when attempting to integrate research evidence into practice. Their seven-stage model consists of:

1 reception/acquisition stage, when practitioners search for and find research that is relevant to their practice;
2 cognition stage, when the practitioner critically evaluates the research evidence;
3 reference stage, when the practitioner begins to integrate theoretical and research evidence into practice;
4 effort stage, when the practitioner applies the research evidence to his or her specific practice and to specific clients;
5 adoption stage, when knowledge gleaned from research evidence is applied to enhance, develop or change existing practices;
6 implementation stage, when research evidence is more thoroughly integrated to underpin practice;
7 impact stage, the final stage, when the impact and value of the research evidence is evaluated.

Knott and Wildavsky's model can be seen as a forerunner of the EBP process. It outlines stages of thinking but does not really give clear guidance to the therapist struggling to develop the skills or ways of critical thinking that underpin EBP. Nor does it deal with the changes required to develop the skills of EBP in either the individual therapist or the institutional culture.

Brown and Rodger (1999) reviewed a number of research utilization models that had been developed and applied within healthcare settings. All of the models attempted to bridge the perceived gap between research and practice. However, some models focused on individual activity whilst others were aimed at team and institutional activities. All models involved the critique and application of research

into practice. For some, application was refined into clinical guidelines and protocols or procedures to guide practice. Some models assumed knowledge of and
a commitment to the use and critique of research evidence, whilst other models
specifically included a stage of skill development as part of the model. Some of
the models have been further refined or researched in practice. All of the models
stressed the importance of a supportive work culture and environment and the
availability of resources to ensure the success of the research utilization process.
No one model appears to provide all of the answers to becoming an evidence-
based occupational therapist. However, there are a number of important messages
about skills development and the need for resources and a supportive environment that give us food for thought as we continue to explore the best ways to
manage the change to EBOT.

Given the emphasis on dissemination and implementation activities to promote
the utilization of research findings within many of the research utilization models,
it seems appropriate to comment on the systematic review by Bero *et al.* (1998) of
interventions to promote the implementation of research findings. Bero *et al.*
found that research studies implied that some research utilization activities were
more effective than others. Activities that had limited effectiveness in changing
practice included passive dissemination activities such as the publication of critically appraised papers (CAPs), an activity that is growing in popularity within
OT journals (e.g. the *Australian Occupational Therapy Journal*). Activities shown to
be most effective were those that involved active participation (e.g. interactive
workshops) or multifaceted interventions, where a number of activities were used
in combination (e.g. evidence-based audit, development of practice guides and
interactive teaching sessions). However, Bero *et al.* concluded that the evidence
for any intervention was mixed and that an understanding of the principles of the
management of change was vital if research utilization and implementation was
to be successful.

Craik and Rappolt (2003) developed the Theory of Research Utilization Enhancement in Occupational Therapy and the Model of Research Utilization in Occupational Therapy from a grounded theory study of the ways elite occupational
therapists working in stroke rehabilitation used research within their practice. The
theory extends and applies Knott and Wildavsky's (1980) stages of knowledge utilization and encompasses a particular model of decision-making (the Occupational
Performance Process Model; Fearing *et al.* 1997). Two of the key findings of the
study are the importance of reflective self-analysis and discussion with peers and
students as tools for linking experiential and research knowledge. Whilst the theory
and model have much to recommend them, the focus on one clinical decision-
making model restricts their usefulness, as does the assumption of personal moti-
vation to be an evidence-based practitioner and to acquire the skills of EBP.

As we have seen, the various models of research utilization have much to offer
in terms of identifying activities to encourage the change to EBOT. However, none
of these models explores how the individual therapist makes the challenging
and critical decision to change and to become an evidence-based occupational
therapist.

Using change management to develop an evidence-based culture

Changing to an evidence-based way of thinking can involve considerable challenges. EBP challenges existing practice to ensure that it is the most appropriate intervention; this can be an uncomfortable process. Changing to EBP also involves the development, or redevelopment, of skills in research and information finding in order to be able to find and appraise the evidence, which might also be challenging. Some therapists will be enthusiastic and ready for this challenge whilst others will be resistant and reluctant to change or to challenge existing practice based on long-held beliefs. Successful change means that everybody, from enthusiast to resister, is accommodated. The key to successful change is to acknowledge these differences and to work with them. Planning the process of change is essential. To plan successfully one must understand both the stages involved in change and the different responses individuals have to change.

Perhaps the best known and most commonly used model of change is the transtheoretical model of change of Prochaska and DiClemente (1982; Prochaska *et al.* 1992). Whilst this was initially developed as a model to explain the process of change for people with addictive behaviours, this model has much wider applications in helping us to understand the process needed to change behaviours and to become an evidence-based occupational therapist (Chilvers *et al.* 2002; McCluskey & Cusick 2002).

Prochaska and DiClemente identified five stages in the process of change. These stages and their application to evidence-based OT are summarized in Table 7.3. This shows that the transtheoretical model can be used to outline the actions required to become an evidence-based occupational therapist.

However, it is also worth bearing in mind what Rogers (1983) identified about the ways different individuals might approach change, and how this can be harnessed in the development of an evidence-based culture. Rogers (1983) identified five different types of individual regarding approaches to change:

■ innovators – constantly looking for ways to improve and develop practice, who will be prepared to drive the development of EBOT forwards;
■ early adopters – will be the next to take up the EBOT challenge and who will be enthusiastic for change and development;
■ early majority – tend to want to stay with the status quo and will be somewhat sceptical of the change to EBOT but will support the change, once they have confidence in the value of EBOT and perceive that change is inevitable;
■ late majority – reluctant to change;
■ laggards – have change forced upon them.

It is important to identify where individuals are in their approaches to change and to work with them wherever they are in the process of change. The innovators and the early adopters will be valuable in getting EBOT started, but the early majority will need to be convinced of the value of EBOT if any changes are to be maintained. The late majority, and particularly the laggards, will need much more

Table 7.3 The stages of change and their application to evidence-based occupational therapy (EBOT).

Stage	Behaviours	EBOT activity
Precontemplation	No intention to change. No awareness of a need to change. May feel anxious and defensive. May feel coerced into EBOT activity.	No EBOT activity. No attempt is made to reflect on practice. Tendency to rely on experiential evidence to guide practice. Supervision might be used as a way of presenting EBOT as a concept worth thinking about.
Contemplation	Are aware of the need to change. Ambivalent about changing behaviours. Needing to weigh up the pros and cons of action.	Demonstrating an interest in EBOT. Asking questions about EBOT. Acknowledging that experiential evidence might not be sufficient to guide practice. Need an opportunity to discuss the pros and cons of EBOT.
Preparation	Intending to take action to change behaviour in the near future.	Identifying the skills required for EBOT and going on courses to develop these skills (e.g. library and searching skills; appraisal skills). Beginning to read critically appraised papers (CAPs). Support is needed to encourage the transition to action.
Action	Modification and change in behaviour and thinking in order to overcome problem. Overt behavioural change. Requires considerable commitment and effort.	Adopting an evidence-based approach to practice. Developing questions. Reading and appraising research papers. Reflecting on practice, articulating experiential evidence and exploring research evidence in order to change outdated behaviours. Support from colleagues and managers is required for action to be maintained.
Maintenance	Working to prevent relapse and to make changes permanent. Consolidating gains. Continued action is required – not a time to rest on one's laurels!	Ongoing and regular use of EBOT activities. Regular reading of a range of journals. Regular question development and literature searching. Active membership of a journal club. Ongoing support and use of supervision is needed to ensure that EBOT becomes a permanent way of thinking and working.

direct intervention and guidance to encourage their acceptance of EBOT; this may have to be linked to appraisal and the establishing of learning contracts to encourage the development of EBOT skills.

It is evident, both from the transtheoretical model and from the work on research utilization, that the change to evidence-based OT is both an individual and an institutional process.

Developing an evidence-based culture

Fundamental to the development of EBOT is the development of a culture that supports an evidence-based approach to practice. Gray (2001, p. 36) suggests that an organization, or department, with an evidence-based culture has 'an obsession with finding, appraising and using research-based knowledge in decision making'. To draw on Cusick's (2001) notion of EBP as asking the 'right' questions, we could develop Gray's definition and suggest that an evidence-based culture facilitates practitioners to ask the 'right' questions about their practice and to answer these questions with the 'right' evidence. Practice settings with evidence-based cultures should be challenging places to work; they should expect practitioners to evaluate their practice and to be able to support and justify their actions using suitable evidence. To do this, however, requires support, evidence-based skills and evidence-based activities.

Support is needed from the management of any team of occupational therapists who are attempting to develop an evidence-based culture. Managers must support moves to challenge and change outdated and redundant practices. EBOT requires access to library and IT resources. It requires time, both to develop skills and to engage in the evidence-based process. Managers need to be prepared to release funding and allow time and space in busy work schedules.

A multifaceted approach to developing an evidence-based culture has been highlighted in the research on research utilization. The variety of evidence-based activities might include:

- Using local opinion leaders to talk to the staff team about EBOT;
- Developing links with local academic institutions, so that they might act as mentors;
- Using interactions with students as a way of challenging practice;
- Running workshops on EBOT skills;
- Establishing a journal club;
- Establishing action learning sets to explore current and future practice;
- Carrying out evidence-based audit of current practice;
- Developing practice guidelines.

The benefits of EBP have been outlined by Rosenberg and Donald (1995). These benefits are presented in Table 7.4. Whilst EBP is still too new within OT to have been evaluated, there is evidence from medicine of its effectiveness (Bennett *et al.* 1987; Shin *et al.* 1993).

Table 7.4 Benefits of practising evidence-based healthcare.

For individual practitioners
▪ Enables practitioners to upgrade their knowledge-base routinely
▪ Improves practitioners' critical understanding of research methods and practice
▪ Improves confidence in management decisions
▪ Improves computer literacy and data searching skills
▪ Improves reading habits

For departments
▪ Gives a framework for group problem-solving and teaching
▪ Enables everyone to contribute to the team

For patients
▪ More effective use of resources
▪ Better communication with patients about the rationale behind intervention proposals

Activity

▪ Identify where you are in relation to Prochaska and DiClemente's stages of change; what actions do you need to undertake to develop or maintain your EBOT behaviour?
▪ Are you an innovator or a laggard? Spend some time reflecting on where you might locate yourself in Rogers' five approaches to change in terms of EBOT.
▪ Identify which of the barriers to becoming an evidence-based occupational therapist (outlined above) are most applicable to you and your work setting – a collaborative approach to this activity might be useful.
▪ Outline the strategies most suitable to overcome the barriers you have identified.
▪ Discuss the barriers and strategies with your line manager.
▪ Develop a strategy for becoming a more evidence-based occupational therapist.

Further reading

The following references will give the reader more scope to explore the complexities of implementing evidence-based practice within OT and beyond.

Alnervik, A. & Svidén, G. (1996) On clinical reasoning: patterns of reflection on practice. *Occupational Therapy Journal of Research* **16**(2), 98–110.

Castle, A. (1996) Developing an ethos of reflective practice for continuing professional development. *British Journal of Therapy and Rehabilitation* **3**(7), 358–359.

Dunning, M., Abi-Aad, G., Gilbert, D., Gillam, S. & Livett, H. (1998) *Turning Evidence into Everyday Practice.* London: King's Fund.

Fish, D., Twinn, S. & Purr, B. (1991) *Promoting Reflection: Improving the Supervision of Practice Health Visiting and Initial Teacher Training.* West London Institute of Higher Education: West London Press.

Heasell, S. (1996) The risky economics of evidence-based medicine. *Health Care Risk Report* November, 22–24.

Hicks, N.R. & Mant, J. (1997) Using the evidence: putting the research into practice. *British Journal of Midwifery* **5**(7), 396–399.

Hunt, M. (1987) The process of translating research findings into nursing practice. *Journal of Advanced Nursing* **12**, 101–110.

Landry, D.W. & Mathews, M. (1998) Economic evaluation of occupational therapy: where are we at? *Canadian Journal of Occupational Therapy* **65**(3), 160–167.

McCluskey, A. & Cusick, A. (2002) Strategies for introducing evidence-based practice and changing clinician behaviour: a manager's toolbox. *Australian Occupational Therapy Journal* **49**, 63–70.

Newdick, C. (1996) The status of guidelines. *Health Care Risk Report* October, 14–15.

Plastow, N. (2006) Implementing evidence-based practice: a model for change. *International Journal of Therapy and Rehabilitation* **13**(10), 464–469.

Rappolt, S. (2003) The role of professional expertise in evidence-based occupational therapy. *American Journal of Occupational Therapy* **57**(5), 589–593.

Schön, D. (1983) *The Reflective Practitioner*. New York: Basic Books.

Stewart, R. (1998) More art than science? *Health Service Journal* 26 March, 28–29.

Walshe, K. (1996) Evidence-based health care – brave new world? *Health Care Risk Report* March, 16–18.

8: Carrying out a review of the evidence

Systematic reviews have already been discussed in detail in Chapter 4. The aim of this chapter is to explore the process of conducting a review of the evidence for a specific topic or evidence-based question. All preregistration occupational therapy (OT) students are involved in research projects at some stage in their OT education. Many students opt to undertake a review project. Some students are required to develop critically appraised topics (CATs) as part of their studies. Equally, many OT teams may decide to carry out a thorough review of the evidence for their practice area for a number of reasons: as a way of demonstrating the value of their service; as part of an evidence-based audit; or as part of the process of developing guidelines for their practice area. This chapter will provide a step-by-step guide to help anyone about to embark on undertaking a review of the evidence for their chosen topic.

This chapter does not aim to explain how to carry out a thorough Cochrane-standard systematic review; this level of review is beyond the scope of any pre-registration student project or OT departmental review. The type of reviews that are within the scope of this chapter should, however, still be covered by the definition of systematic reviews given by the UK's National Health Service Centre for Reviews and Dissemination (NHS CRD 2001, p. i) as reviews that 'locate, appraise and synthesise evidence from scientific studies'.

Just as carrying out an empirical research project requires planning and careful adherence to a logical research process, so carrying out a review is guided by a clear and logical review process. Box 8.1 gives an overview of the review process.

The remainder of this chapter will discuss each of the stages of the process, with illustrations from a fictional review, in order to give pointers for the successful completion of a review project.

Planning and protocol development

The first, and probably most important, stage of the review process is the planning stage (Box 8.2). This stage may also involve the development of a formal plan, or protocol. This protocol may range from a short summary of the activities to be

Box 8.1 The stages of the review process

■ Planning and protocol development
■ Defining the question
■ Searching for the evidence
■ Selecting the evidence to include in the review
■ Assessing how 'good' the evidence is
■ Extracting the important information
■ Presenting the findings
■ Synthesis of the findings and drawing the review together

Box 8.2 Planning a review

The reviewer is interested in undertaking a review into the value of fatigue management for people experiencing multiple sclerosis (MS)-related fatigue. In order to plan effectively she must understand:

■ **the policy context**
  ● reviewing the National Service Framework (NSF) on Long Term Conditions will provide useful policy background, as will establishing how prevalent both MS and MS-related fatigue are within the population, and the nature of the MS population receiving interventions for fatigue
■ **the OT context**
  ● what is the role of OT when working with people with MS and MS-related fatigue?
■ **the nature of the intervention and problem**
  ● what exactly are MS and MS-related fatigue?
  ● is MS-related fatigue different from other forms of fatigue?
  ● how is MS-related fatigue managed?
  ● what does a fatigue management programme consist of; which professionals are involved; is it individual or group-based?
■ **the range of research**
  ● fatigue management is an intervention and, therefore, should be researched using RCTs, but what would such an RCT look like?
  ● fatigue is a subjective experience, so should also be researched using qualitative methods; what can this type of research tell us and how might a qualitative study be carried out?
■ **possible outcomes**
  ● how has fatigue been measured?
  ● what is the range of the potential outcome measures that might be used in research studies?

undertaken at each stage of the review to a detailed outline that forms a formal part of the assessment process. The idea of the protocol, and the importance of the planning phase, is to ensure that the review has a clear focus and that the reviewer has a sound understanding not only of the review process but also of the background to the topic under review.

Before the review question can be articulated it is important to have a sound understanding of the topic to be reviewed. This will include establishing the background in a number of areas including:

- the policy context;
- the OT context;
- the nature of the intervention or problem;
- the range of research possibilities;
- the possible outcomes being researched.

Exploring the policy and professional OT context of the problem is important as it will establish a clear rationale for conducting a review into the particular topic. Having a clear understanding of the intervention or problem will mean that the reviewer will have an understanding of how the intervention has been used, whether other professionals are involved and who the potential research participants might be.

Scrutinizing the potential range of research methodologies used to explore this intervention or problem will help in planning the scope of the review both in terms of the methodologies of the review and also the viability of the review. Important questions to ask here include whether clinical trials – randomized controlled trials (RCTs) and controlled clinical trials (CCTs) – or qualitative research will provide the most useful evidence for the review. The potential viability of any review must also be considered at this stage by ensuring that sufficient published research is available on the topic to be able to complete a review. The author recommends that her students are aware of at least six published and relevant research studies when they are planning their review protocols.

The final background area to be explored at the planning stage is the potential outcomes or ways that the intervention or problem has been measured. Defining the outcome part of any PICO (problem, intervention, comparison, outcome) evidence-based question is often the hardest, and becomes even harder when the reviewer has no clear idea of what measures have been used by the researchers.

Defining the question

Having established the background to the topic area, the reviewer should have a clearer idea of how to define, or articulate, the review question, which will then provide a clear framework for the review (Box 8.3). As Alderson *et al.* (2004) point out, the question provides the direction for all of the review's tasks. A poorly defined, or vague, question will result in a review that is of poor quality and of little value to the evidence-based occupational therapist. It might be worth reviewing what Chapter 1 had to say on asking evidence-based questions.

Box 8.3 Possible review questions

Review questions can cover a number of areas:

- assessments
- goal setting
- therapy and interventions
- individual experiences

Whilst the MS-related fatigue review is primarily about therapy/intervention, a number of potential review questions could be suggested:

- assessments – in clients experiencing MS-related fatigue, what is the most effective tool for assessing and measuring MS-related fatigue?
- goal setting – at what point in the disease process should clients with MS be involved in a fatigue management programme?
- therapy and interventions – what evidence is there for the effectiveness of a fatigue management programme on the reduction and management of fatigue in clients with MS?
- individual experiences – when planning a fatigue management programme, what can be learnt from the experiences of people with MS-related fatigue about the impact of fatigue on their lives, and how they manage their illness?

Searching for the evidence

A basic search and review of the literature will have been carried out as part of the planning phase of the review. The search phase involves a much more thorough and rigorous search of the available literature and should consist of a number of aspects:

- defining the search;
- searching the databases;
- hand searching;
- citation tracking.

It may also involve:

- contacting researchers and authors;
- searching the grey literature.

However, these two aspects are often inappropriate for preregistration students' review projects.

Defining the search

Chapter 2 discussed how to develop a search strategy. The first and, again, most important part of the search is to ensure that the search strategy is clearly defined, so that the search is thorough and rigorous and the outcomes of the search can

Box 8.4 Developing the search strategy

A search strategy can be based on the following aspects:
- types of research;
- participants in the research;
- interventions included in the research;
- outcomes to be measured.

In terms of the review on the effectiveness of fatigue management this might mean:

- **types of research:**
  - RCTs and CCTs
- **participants in the research:**
  - people with a clinical diagnosis of MS
- **interventions included in the research:**
  - fatigue management programmes
  - either group or individual
  - carried out by occupational therapists, either alone or in combination with other healthcare professionals
- **outcomes to be measured:**
  - fatigue management rating scales
  - self-efficacy for fatigue management scales

be recorded and included in the review report. The areas to be defined in the search strategy are outlined in Box 8.4. These areas can then be used to identify the actual search terms to be used.

Searching the databases

As discussed in Chapter 2, it is important to search more than one database. It is also important to have a clear rationale for the choice of particular databases to be included, and not just to search all databases that one has access to. The choice of database will depend both on the nature of the problem and also the types of research to be included. Searching the Cochrane Library or OTseeker would be inappropriate for a review focusing on qualitative research, but would be vital for a review of effectiveness that included RCTs.

It is important that you record all searches, and the number of 'hits' at each stage of the search. This information is important in ensuring the transparency of your review. The records of your searches and their outputs should be included as appendix material for the final report.

Hand searching

Hand searching, as the name suggests, involves going through hard copies of relevant journals page by page in order to identify any potentially relevant papers. Whilst databases give access to a vast amount of literature, they are only as good (or useful) as the indexers and the terms they are given, and any database may not include all of the potentially relevant journals. MEDLINE, for example, has very limited coverage of the OT literature. Hand searching is important as it allows the reviewer to identify papers that might otherwise have been missed. Hand searching is, however, time consuming, but it is effective (Hopewell *et al.* 2004). Before beginning to hand search, reviewers must ask themselves two important questions:

■ What journals should I hand search?
■ How far back should I go?

The choice of journals to be hand searched should be governed by relevance rather than logistics or pragmatic considerations. Journals should not be selected for hand searching simply because you have easy access to them. Access to journals online means that hand searching can often be done from the comfort of your desk, rather than spending valuable time visiting a number of different libraries. However, the reviewer must think carefully about the scope of any hand search and the breadth of journals to be included and be prepared with a clear rationale for which journals might, or might not, be usefully hand searched.

Citation tracking

Citation tracking is the technical term for checking the reference lists of any relevant research papers to see if you can identify any new research articles or other papers that you have not identified in any other searches. This is a useful exercise as, not only might it give you access to a paper you had otherwise missed, it might also help you to identify key studies in your particular field. Key studies are easily identified; they are the papers that everyone refers back to. They may have started the research in the area or have developed a useful measurement tool or research methodology, which other researchers have then used or refined.

Citation searching is a useful variation of citation tracking. You may have noticed that when you identify a particular article using a database search there is usually a link identified as 'Find Citing Articles'. If the paper appears to be particularly useful (a key study) it might be worth following this link to identify other papers that have cited this particular study.

Selecting the evidence to include in the review

Having carried out your thorough and rigorous search, you will have identified a number of papers that are potentially of value to your review. But are they all of value, should they all be included in the review? The next stage in the review process is to sift through all of these identified studies and decide which ones meet the specific criteria of your study.

Table 8.1 Examples of inclusion and exclusion criteria.

	Inclusion criteria	Exclusion criteria
Participants	Clinical diagnosis of MS	Clinical diagnoses of chronic fatigue or other non-MS-related fatigue
Interventions	Fatigue management groups Fatigue management individual programmes	
Outcomes	MS fatigue rating scales MS-specific self-efficacy scales	Non-MS-specific fatigue scales
Type of research	RCTs and CCTs	
Other		
Language	English language	Non-English language
Publication date	1995 onwards	Pre-1995

As part of the planning process you will have identified your inclusion and exclusion criteria. Now is the time to apply those criteria to identify the studies that will make up your review of the evidence. The studies that you exclude should not be discarded, they may provide useful background information; a list of all the excluded studies, and the reasons for their exclusion, should be included as an appendix within your final report. Having clear inclusion and exclusion criteria ensures that your choice of studies is transparent, and not based on personal bias or chance identification of a number of possibly interesting papers.

The main inclusion criteria will focus around the aspects of your review question, in terms of the intervention, the clients and the outcomes, as well as the types of research studies to be included. Possible inclusion and exclusion criteria are illustrated in Table 8.1. You may also decide to refine your material for practical reasons by including only English-language papers or to ensure that only current evidence is included. You may also decide to have specific exclusions to avoid confusion or to ensure the focus of your review.

Assessing how 'good' the evidence is

Having identified the studies to be included in the review it is important to assess the research rigour of each study. This process is known as quality assessment. Any review is only as good as the rigour of each of the component studies, otherwise it will be a case of GIGO (garbage in and garbage out; Greenhalgh 2006).

Chapters 3 and 5 discussed the key factors to consider in terms of the rigour of both RCTs and qualitative research and also discussed how to critically appraise these types of studies. It is important to note here that critical appraisal and quality assessment are NOT the same. There are two key differences between critical appraisal and quality assessment. The process of quality assessment focuses solely on the research rigour of the study and also aims to produce some form of overall score of the research rigour, so that studies can be compared in terms of the rigour, or strength, of the evidence. Critical appraisal looks beyond rigour to include the relevance of the study to a particular setting and does not include a scoring system for the strength of the evidence. It is, therefore, important that the checklists used for critical appraisal are not mistaken for the tools used in quality assessment.

A number of checklists and tools have been designed to assess the quality of RCTs (Moher *et al.* 1995; Jadad *et al.* 1996). One possible RCT quality assessment tool that is readily accessible is the PEDro Scale, which is used on both PEDro and OTseeker. This has been shown to be a robust tool and is beginning to be used in published OT reviews. Quality assessment of qualitative research studies is more complex and contentious, and fewer checklists and tools exist, although the strategy developed by Spencer *et al.* (2003) might have some value.

Once you have carried out the quality assessment of each of the potential studies, you may decide to review your inclusion criteria and to exclude any studies that might be deemed poor quality based on their quality assessment scores.

Extracting the important information

Once you have identified the good-quality studies that you will include in your review you then need to decide which pieces of information from each paper are important and to collect all of this information together in an organized format. This process is known as 'data extraction'.

The process of data extraction involves recording information onto some form of proforma or template; this information can then be used to structure the various tables that will present the findings of the review in the finished report (see below). Examples of data extraction forms can be found in the 'Reviews Guidance' published by the UK's NHS Centre for Reviews and Dissemination (NHS CRD 2001), but reviewers often feel the need to design their own data extraction forms to meet the specific needs of their review. It is worth noting that separate data extraction forms will be needed for different types of research.

Table 8.2 gives examples of some of the types of headings a data extraction form might include. It is worthwhile pilot-testing the data extraction form on a few of your research studies, to ensure that the form works and that it enables you to identify and record all the relevant information from each research paper.

Table 8.2 Examples of data extraction headings.

Data to be extracted	Notes for reviewer	Data extracted
Title of paper		
Author		
Source/publication		
Date of publication		
Study objectives		
Type of study		
Participants		
Sample information		
Interventions		
Outcomes measured		
Results		
Quality assessment score		

Presenting the findings

The Results section of the review report consists of a series of tables giving:

■ the results of the search, in terms of number of hits and the number of included and excluded studies;
■ a summary of the key points drawn from the included studies.

These tables should include an overview of the research methodology and quality assessment scores for each of the included studies. Other tables should give details of the analysis and results of the various studies. It is your job, as the reviewer, to decide how to present your review findings in table form and to ensure that the tables give a clear overview of the information from the various studies. This will enable the reader to follow and assess your synthesis of the material and the conclusions that you draw. It is also useful to provide a narrative that describes to the reader exactly what each of the tables is attempting to show.

Before you prepare the tables for your final report it is worth spending some time looking at published reviews to see how they have presented their findings and the ways they have used both tables and narrative to present the information clearly.

Synthesis of the findings and drawing the review together

Presenting the findings of the review in a series of tables does not really provide a thorough answer to the review question; for this the findings must be compared and synthesized, so that a summary can be prepared that will answer the review question. Meta-analysis provides a statistical synthesis of the findings of the studies included in a review. However, meta-analysis is beyond the scope of the preregistration review project and many studies of OT interventions are too heterogeneous to permit this level of analysis to be carried out.

Narrative synthesis gives the reviewer the opportunity to draw the review together and to comment on the quality of the evidence that has been reviewed. The narrative synthesis should usually include the following areas:

- discussion of the methodological quality;
- comparison of the various studies.

Discussion of the methodological quality

The value of the quality assessment of the various included studies is to highlight the strength of the evidence provided by each of the studies. A high-quality assessment score indicates strong evidence, whilst a lower score indicates weaker evidence. It is, therefore, important to give an overview and a commentary on the methodological quality and rigour of the various studies and to highlight whether there is high-quality evidence to support the intervention or topic being reviewed.

Comparison of the various studies

How the synthesis and comparison of the various studies is structured will depend both upon the nature of the review question and also on the types of included studies. It may, however, be relevant to comment on:

- similarities and differences in the study samples;
- similarities and differences in the study designs;
- similarities and differences in the way the intervention was carried out;
- similarities and differences in the outcomes that were measured and the outcome measurements that were used.

This will give the reader a sense of how comparable the studies are, and the scope of the evidence that is being reviewed.

It is also important to comment on the findings of the different studies and particularly the statistical analysis and outcomes, and to compare and comment on any differences between the different findings. It is important to note whether high-quality studies achieve statistically significant results, or if only the low-quality studies have statistically significant results, which might call the real significance of these findings into question. It is also important to review how many of the studies show significant results as opposed to no significant results. If there are a number of studies that did not achieve statistically significant results this will indicate that there is, at best, ambivalent evidence in support of the intervention and at worst no evidence to support the intervention.

In a review that focuses on qualitative evidence, the reviewer must attempt to synthesize the findings of the various studies using the themes that have emerged from them. This may involve identifying where studies have found similar themes as well as exploring the range of themes across the various studies. The process of synthesis of qualitative findings is being developed and has been variously described as meta-ethnography, meta-synthesis and meta-narrative (Greenhalgh *et al.* 2005).

The goal of the synthesis is to provide the reader with a clear understanding of whether there is evidence to answer the review question and what the answer to the question might be. The reviewer should provide a summary that can address the review question, indicating whether there is evidence, strong evidence, no evidence or ambivalent evidence to answer the review question. The reviewer should also highlight any weaknesses within the review process and indicate possible directions for future research.

Hopefully this chapter has clarified the process of conducting a review project, given you pointers to tools for the process and inspired you to carry out your own review of the research literature relating to a topic or intervention that particularly interests you.

Further reading

Alderson, P., Green, S. & Higgins, J. (2004) *Cochrane Reviewers' Handbook 4.2.2*. Chichester: John Wiley & Sons.

Dickson, R. (2005) Systematic reviews. In: Hamer, S. & Collinson, G. (eds) *Achieving Evidence-based Practice*. Edinburgh: Baillière Tindall, pp. 43–62.

Greenhalgh, T., Robert, G., Macfarlane, F., Bate, P., Kyriakidou, O. & Peacock, R. (2005) Storylines of research in diffusion of innovation: a meta-narrative approach to systematic reviews. *Social Science and Medicine* **61**, 417–430.

Massy-Westropp, N. & Masters, M. (2003) Doing systematic reviews in an occupational therapy department. *British Journal of Occupational Therapy* **66**(9), 427–430.

NHS CRD (2001) *Undertaking Systematic Reviews of Research on Effectiveness: CRD's Guidance to those Carrying out or Commissioning Reviews*. CRD Report 4, 2nd edn. York: Centre for Reviews and Dissemination, University of York.

Petticrew, M. & Roberts, H. (2006) *Systematic Reviews in the Social Sciences*. Oxford: Blackwell Publishing.

9: Developing and using guidelines for practice

If evidence-based practice is about giving practitioners the tools to 'do the right things right' (Gray 2001), then guidelines are key tools for the evidence-based occupational therapist. Guidelines can be seen as the end product of an evidence-based approach, where evidence is reviewed and synthesized to improve intervention and occupational therapy (OT) practice not only for an individual client but also for a group of clients with a particular problem or need. Guidelines aim to map out interventions and intervention processes for particular conditions. Guidelines have been used to underpin and outline good practice and are often used as tools within the audit process. Guidelines can be developed at both local and national levels.

This chapter will give the evidence-based occupational therapist the tools to look critically at any guideline. It will also explain ways of successfully implementing guidelines within the practice setting and will outline how the evidence-based occupational therapist can go about developing her or his own guidelines for a particular practice.

What are guidelines?

Clinical guidelines have been defined as:

> systematically developed statements to assist practitioner decisions about appropriate health care for specific clinical circumstances
>
> (Thomas *et al.* 1999, p. 2).

They are seen as tools to help managers and practitioners decide about the process of interventions. Guidelines provide principles upon which to base interventions and service delivery, and against which the standards and quality of interventions and service delivery can be assessed and measured. Austin and Herbert (1995) outline the purpose of clinical guidelines as:

- Collecting sound evidence of the efficacy of a pattern of behaviour, for example RCTs;
- Providing expert knowledge in an agreed and easy to use format;
- Making knowledge accessible to therapists when they need it;

■ Supporting intervention decision-making;
■ Supporting care plan negotiation between client and therapist;
■ Raising the standards of care;
■ Supporting management functions, especially contracting and budgeting.

The goal of any guideline is to improve the quality of health and social care. However, in the past guidelines were rarely evidence-based. They were drawn from a synthesis of current best practice, consensus views of practitioners and expert discussion.

In the current climate of evidence-based health and social care, there is a need for more rigorous, systematic and evidence-based guidelines (Mann 1996). These *clinical guidelines* need to be based on current best evidence of effectiveness. Only where evidence is of poor quality, or absent, should expert and professional opinion be used as evidence. These guidelines should focus on specific interventions with specific client groups, much as the evidence-based questions discussed in Chapter 1 have a specific problem, intervention and outcome focus. Clinical guidelines should be based, if possible, on systematic reviews of the relevant evidence. Where clinical guidelines differ from systematic reviews is that a clinical guideline will develop and outline clear recommendations and principles upon which practice and interventions can be based. Systematic reviews give both the statistical and clinical significance of the findings, but do not attempt to go beyond these or make recommendations about interventions.

Before we explore guidelines further, it might be useful to define some terms that are commonly used when discussing guidelines. The terms *protocol, care pathway* and *guideline* are often used interchangeably. However, these terms have different meanings and different purposes.

Protocols are 'rigid statements allowing little or no flexibility or variation. A protocol sets out a precise sequence of activities to be adhered to in the management of a specific clinical condition' (Broughton & Rathbone 2003, p. 2). Thus a protocol is a prescriptive set of rules for a particular task or situation.

Care pathways give a picture of the client's journey through a particular care situation and can allow for change and flexibility. 'An integrated care pathway is a multidisciplinary outline of anticipated care, placed in an appropriate timeframe, to help a patient with a specific condition or set of symptoms move progressively through a clinical experience to positive outcomes' (Middelton *et al.* 2003, p. 1).

Guidelines, as we have already seen, attempt to define best and most effective practice but are recommendations, which still allow the practitioner to use professional judgment when deciding the best intervention for a particular client.

The growth of guidelines

Since the publication of two key documents – *A First Class Service: Quality in the New NHS* (Department of Health 1998) and *Modernising Social Services*

(Department of Health 1998) – the development and use of guidelines has been an integral part of health and social care policy in the UK. This has led to the establishment of both NICE (National Institute for Health and Clinical Excellence) and SCIE (Social Care Institute for Excellence) and the publication of numerous evidence-based guidelines to ensure best practice in health and social care interventions. SIGN (the Scottish Intercollegiate Guidelines Network) and NZGG (New Zealand Guidelines Group) are a few of the other groups producing national guidelines for practice.

One of the drawbacks of national guidelines is that they tend to take a broad-brush approach and rarely look specifically at interventions or activities of particular professional groups, such as OT; hence, OT-specific guidelines are relatively rare. An excellent example of a guideline, which has been instrumental in improving the delivery and quality of OT practice, is the work done in Canada developing client-centred practice in OT (Canadian Association of Occupational Therapists 1991a; Law 1998). Whilst Thomas *et al.* (1999) found no evidence for the use of clinical guidelines within OT, the College of Occupational Therapists (2004) has sought to encourage occupational therapists in the UK to produce specific OT guidelines for practice, an example of which are the guidelines for rheumatology produced by the National Association of Rheumatology Occupational Therapists (2003). Evidence-based occupational therapists will have to be creative in their searching in order to locate guidelines that might have specific relevance for their area of practice.

Using guidelines to improve practice

Greenhalgh (2006) points out that policy-makers, managers and academics love guidelines, because they present a clear, if idealized, concept of best practice. Less enamoured of guidelines are front-line practitioners, because they are the ones who have to balance the ideals with the realities of best practice within the context of local service constraints. What factors can facilitate the successful implementation of a guideline?

The process of implementing the principles outlined within a clinical guideline will require not only individual but institutional commitment to change. A team approach is necessary, as guidelines are unlikely to affect the practice of just a single professional group. Management support is required, and a formal system of review must be established to audit the effectiveness and effects of the implementation of the guideline.

A number of factors have been found to influence whether practitioners follow a guideline (Grol *et al.* 1998); they include whether the guideline:

- is uncontroversial;
- is evidence based;
- contains explicit recommendations;
- requires little or no change to existing practice.

Grimshaw and Russell (1993) also found that the most effective guidelines were developed at the local level by the people who were going to use them and introduced with specific educational and dissemination activities. The importance of locally developed guidelines does not mean that the national guidelines produced by NICE and others will not be effectively implemented. Rather it means that when attempting to implement any guideline the local practitioners should be directly involved in the creation of a development and implementation plan for the guideline at local level, thus ensuring that the guideline is able to accommodate the local practice context.

The legal implications of guidelines

Guidelines provide an overview of what best practice should consist of. As such they are rarely mandatory; they do not replace the individual professional's responsibility and duty of care to provide best practice. A guideline cannot replace clinical reasoning and professional judgment, in consultation with the client, about the best and most appropriate intervention. If, however, a guideline is in place and the practitioner decides to deviate from the guideline, this decision must be recorded appropriately in the client's notes or records. McClarey and Thompson (2000) note that any health or social care professional who decides not to follow a guideline must provide evidence that the actions taken were acceptable professional practice. Whilst the duty of care rests with the individual professional, local management also has a duty to provide the appropriate resources to allow practitioners to deliver the interventions as outlined by the guideline.

Appraising guidelines

The questions used to appraise and review a guideline can be divided into two areas:

- the rigour of the review content and presentation;
- the applicability and usefulness of the review.

Table 9.1 outlines the questions. Inspiration for the development of these appraisal questions has been drawn from a number of sources including Greenhalgh (2006) and Strauss *et al.* (2005).

How rigorous are the guidelines?

Does the guideline have a clear scope and purpose?

As with any evidence-based question, the focus of any guideline should be clearly stated and should provide not only a clear focus for the guideline but also provide

Table 9.1 Questions to ask when critically appraising guidelines.

How rigorous are the guidelines?
■ Does the guideline have a clear scope and purpose?
■ Were all appropriate stakeholders included in the guideline development process?
■ Have all relevant studies/sources been reviewed and evaluated?
■ Has the evidence been appropriately synthesized?
■ Are the recommendations suitably graded and linked to specific evidence?
■ Do the guidelines include recommendations for regular review and updating?

How will these guidelines help me in my work with clients?
■ Are the guidelines relevant to my practice context?
■ Is the guideline flexible?
■ Does the guideline take into account what is acceptable to, affordable by and practical for the context and the clients?
■ Does the guideline include recommendations for dissemination and implementation?

a well-defined scope for the guideline. Thus, it will be clear if the guideline is specific to a particular setting or population. The parameters of the guideline must be clearly articulated so that the reader is clear about who or what the guidelines might be applied to:

■ the population (e.g. how age specific is the guideline?);
■ the setting (e.g. inpatient rather than community);
■ the interventions;
■ the practitioners.

Were all appropriate stakeholders included in the guideline development process?

Producing a guideline is not a task for a solo author but should be a shared task for a guideline development group. This group should consist of all the major stakeholders who might have an interest in the intervention. Stakeholders should range from researchers and others with technical and research skills, through clinicians who will be implementing the guideline, to service users. All of this expertise should be clearly articulated and the involvement of the various stakeholders should be clearly identified. As Swinglehurst (2005) points out, guideline producers should be able to outline the values and guiding principles that underpin their actions and decisions. The importance of the presence of clinicians within the guideline development group was highlighted by the qualitative study by Gabbay and le May (2004) of the implementation of guidelines in practice. Thus the critical reader must be able to identify and assess not only the various stakeholders and their involvement in the process but also the guiding principles that underpin the workings of the guideline's authors.

Have all relevant studies/sources been reviewed and evaluated, and the evidence appropriately synthesized?

As we have seen in previous chapters the nature of 'best' evidence within evidenced-based OT is a matter of considerable debate. Whilst the value of systematic reviews and high-quality RCTs is without question, a sound guideline must also draw on a wide range of evidence sources including qualitative research and expert opinion. How thorough was the search for evidence?

The results of these searches must then be pulled together and synthesized. How adequate is this synthesis? Is the overview of the research findings clear and comprehensive? If expert opinion and consensus have been used, how thorough have the consensus studies been; could the consensus be biased by the strongest voices or have methods been used to ensure that all voices are given equal weighting?

Are the recommendations suitably graded and linked to specific evidence?

Having found and synthesized suitable evidence the guideline developers must then present their recommendations. Is it possible clearly to link particular recommendations with specific research studies? Recommendations should also be graded, but how clear is the grading system?

Do the guidelines include recommendations for regular review and updating?

Developing a rigorous guideline is a time-consuming task. Is the timescale of the guideline's development clear? Based on this information, how up to date is the guideline? Have the developers stated a 'sell-by date' when the guideline might be considered to be out of date or will the guideline be reviewed and updated regularly?

How will these guidelines help me in my work with clients?

Are the guidelines relevant to my practice context?

Go back and look at the scope and parameters of the guideline. How well do these match your particular practice setting? Can you adapt the guideline to suit your particular client group? Grimley Evans (1995) talks of evidence-*biased* medicine and the use of guidelines just because the guideline exists not because it is appropriate to the practice setting.

Is the guideline flexible?

A guideline is not a straightjacket or a rigid protocol; it aims to be exactly what the name suggests, a *guide*. How well does the guideline accommodate the realities of practice, rather than outline an idealized form of best practice? How well does the guideline acknowledge the need to compromise because of financial or other logistical constraints? In an age of limited availability of services does the guideline help to identify the clients who might benefit most?

Does the guideline take into account what is acceptable to, affordable by and practical for the context and the clients?

How well does the guideline accommodate the real world? Are the recommendations too idealistic to be practically possible or acceptable within your professional context?

Does the guideline include recommendations for dissemination and implementation?

As we have seen previously, adopting an evidenced-based approach is not without its barriers. Does the guideline give any indication of how the recommendations might be successfully implemented? Vital to this aspect is the input of clinicians in the guideline development group.

Developing guidelines for practice

It is not the intention of this chapter to give a detailed outline of the process of guideline development; this has been ably done in other places (e.g. New Zealand Guidelines Group 2001; College of Occupational Therapists 2004). It aims, however, to illustrate key aspects of the guideline process. Figure 9.1 gives an overview of the various stages of the guideline development process.

Whilst much of this process is similar to the development and production of a systematic review, the key differences, which will be discussed below, are in three main areas:

- the use of a guideline development group;
- the use of expert opinion and consensus evidence;
- the development and grading of recommendations.

Establishing a guideline development group

Developing a guideline is a complex and time-consuming task, which requires a range of skills from searching for the evidence to developing and grading recommendations for practice. Therefore, to successfully develop a rigorous and credible guideline a guideline development group should be established, which includes all the relevant stakeholders. The range of people and skills needed include:

- someone to chair and lead the group;
- people with search and IT skills;

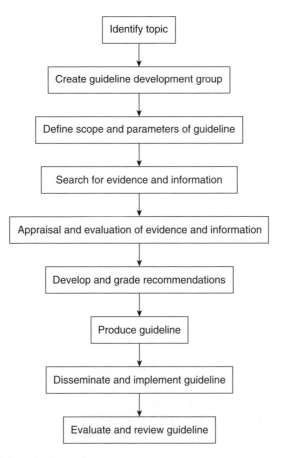

Figure 9.1 The guideline development process.

■ people with research skills;
■ expert practitioners;
■ people with writing skills;
■ administrative and organizational skills;
■ service users.

The group will need to meet initially to develop the plan for the guideline development project and to organize and identify tasks and timescales for the project. The group should meet regularly to ensure that the momentum of the project is maintained.

Collecting expert opinion and consensus evidence

The aim of any guideline is to produce recommendations for practice based on the best available evidence and information. Whilst the 'best' evidence is usually acknowledged to be research evidence, preferably systematic reviews and RCTs, this level of evidence is not always available for OT interventions. Where little or no good-quality research evidence is available the accepted alternative is to seek expert opinion and to establish a consensus, or agreement, amongst a panel of experts on what best practice might be.

The two most commonly used methods of gaining consensus information are the nominal group technique and the Delphi technique (Pope & Mays 2006). Both methods assemble a group of experts, either for meetings and discussions (nominal group) or by questionnaire (Delphi), to share information about best practice and then produce some form of agreed list or overview of what constitutes best practice. Deane *et al.* (2003a, 2003b) have successfully used the Delphi technique to establish an overview of best OT practice for people with Parkinson's disease. However, as Greenhalgh (2006) points out, guideline developers must be wary of paying too much attention to the experts with the most to say or of ignoring the quieter members of the group. Murphy *et al.* (1998) provide useful information about the best ways of using consensus information within guideline development.

Developing and grading recommendations

The search for, and review of, evidence and information, including the consensus information and expert opinion, will have identified what constitutes best practice for the area of interest. This information now has to be synthesized to produce the recommendations for practice that will be the core elements of the guideline.

The development of recommendations is the least evidence-based and often most contentious part of the process, as the guideline development group must agree on the recommendations. Thus developing the recommendations is a blend of the art and science of best practice. Each recommendation must, however, be clearly linked to the appropriate evidence and information that supports its inclusion in the guideline. Recommendations should be clear, objective and precise descriptions of actions or a course of actions, as illustrated in Box 9.1.

Recommendations are usually graded to indicate the strength of the evidence or information on which they are based, thus indicating the type of information that has been used to develop each recommendation. This grading is based upon the appraisal and review of the evidence that forms part of the guideline development process (see Fig. 9.1).

The grading of recommendations is not without debate and differing opinions. The more medically oriented guideline developers, such as SIGN, favour the grading system based upon the evidence-based medicine hierarchy of evidence, whilst the NZGG adopts a broader approach to evidence and looks at the rigour of the research irrespective of its design. Both of these grading systems imply a hierarchy of grades and, therefore, show that some recommendations are based on weaker (however defined) evidence. The College of Occupational Therapists (COT) has adopted a non-hierarchical approach, which indicates the type of evidence but does not imply a rigid hierarchy of levels of evidence. Table 9.2 outlines the various grading systems, to allow the evidence-based occupational therapist to review the relative merits of the three approaches.

Box 9.1 Example of a guideline recommendation

Any person with multiple sclerosis (MS) whose participation in or enjoyment of a leisure or social activity becomes limited should be referred to a specialist neurological rehabilitation service which should:

- identify whether previous activities are still achievable and, if not, help the person consider new activities;
- assess for, and then teach, the skills and techniques that could help achieve these activities;
- if necessary refer the person to local services that might help them establish and continue leisure and social activities.

(National Collaborating Centre for Chronic Conditions 2004)

Activity

- Identify any existing clinical guidelines relevant to your area of intervention and practice.
- Discuss the practicalities of implementing these guidelines with your manager.
- Identify other professional groups who might be affected by the implementation of these guidelines.
- Discuss the practicalities of implementing these guidelines with this multidisciplinary team.
- Establish a strategy for the implementation of the guidelines.
- Establish clear outcomes to be used as measures to assess the impact of the implementation of the clinical guidelines.
- Discuss an audit strategy with your local clinical audit/effectiveness department.
- Implement the guidelines.

Table 9.2 Grading systems for recommendations.

Scottish Intercollegiate Guidelines Network (SIGN 2002) Grades of recommendation

A   At least one meta-analysis, systematic review, or RCT rated as 1++ and directly applicable to the target population; or A systematic review of RCTs or a body of evidence consisting principally of studies rated as 1+, directly applicable to the target population, and demonstrating overall consistency of results

B   A body of evidence including studies rated as 2++, directly applicable to the target population, and demonstrating overall consistency of results; or Extrapolated evidence from studies rated as 1++ or 1+

C   A body of evidence including studies rated as 2+, directly applicable to the target population, and demonstrating overall consistency of results; or Extrapolated evidence from studies rated as 2++

D   Evidence level 3 or 4; or Extrapolated evidence from studies rated as 2+

New Zealand Guidelines Group (2001) Grading for recommendations

A   The recommendation (course of action) is supported by good evidence: The evidence consists of results from studies of strong design for answering the question addressed

B   The recommendation (course of action) is supported by fair evidence: The evidence consists of results from studies of strong design for answering the question addressed but there is some uncertainty attached to the conclusion either because of inconsistencies among the results from the studies or because of minor flaws; or the evidence consists of results from weaker study designs for the question addressed but the results have been confirmed in separate studies and are reasonably consistent. There is fair evidence that the benefits of the course of action being proposed outweigh the harms

C   The recommendation (course of action) is supported by expert opinion only: For some outcomes, trials or studies cannot be or have not been performed and practice is informed only by expert opinion

I   No recommendation can be made because the evidence is insufficient: Evidence for a course of action is lacking, of poor quality or conflicting and the balance of benefits and harms cannot be determined

College of Occupational Therapists (2004) Labels for recommendations when based upon:

A   Scientific studies or trials (the actual results of the studies/trials)

B   Systematic reviews or meta-analysis (a secondary review or analysis of several similar studies/trials)

C   Non-analytical studies, e.g. case studies, observations and reports

D   Published knowledge not based upon scientific studies or trials

E   Expert consensus opinion

Further reading and resources

The following references and resources will allow the reader to explore issues pertinent to the understanding and appraisal of different sources of evidence in more depth.

AGREE (Appraisal of Guidelines Research & Evaluation) Collaboration (http://www. agreecollaboration.org).

College of Occupational Therapists (2004) *Practice Guidelines Development Manual.* London: College of Occupational Therapists.

National Association of Rheumatology Occupational Therapists (2003) *Occupational Therapy Clinical Guidelines for Rheumatology.* London: College of Occupational Therapists (www.cot.org.uk/ members/profpractice/guidelines/intro.php).

National Collaborating Centre for Chronic Conditions (2004) *Multiple Sclerosis: National Clinical Guideline for Diagnosis and Management in Primary and Secondary Care.* London: Royal College of Physicians (http://www.rcplondon.ac.uk/pubs/books/MS/index.asp).

National Guideline Clearinghouse. This US government website contains a database of intervention and practice guidelines (http://www.guideline.gov).

10: Useful resources

This chapter will provide the reader with an annotated list of sources of information and resources that may be helpful in the practice of evidence-based occupational therapy (OT). These resources include:

- indexes and databases;
- websites;
- further reading:
  - books;
  - evidence-based journals and publications;
- useful addresses and other miscellaneous resources.

Every effort has been made to ensure that the information presented here is as up to date as possible. However, the author cannot accept responsibility for errors but does apologize for any oversights! This resource information should be seen as a starting point and readers should make use of the blank spaces in the text to add their own resources to the list, enabling them to build up a personal evidence-based practice resource.

Indexes and databases

In terms of the OT literature, the most comprehensive coverage can probably be found using a combination of CINAHL and AMED. However, background material might be more easily found on ASSIA and MEDLINE. Access to databases is available via two main formats: CD-ROMs and the internet. The tendency, currently, is for libraries to move away from subscriptions to hard copies and CD-ROM copies of databases and to move towards subscriptions via the internet. Databases use a variety of software, such as Ovid and SilverPlatter, which have slightly different search strategies. If possible, the evidence-based occupational therapist should access all databases through the same software, as this makes transferring search skills rather easier. As was highlighted in Chapter 2, databases are only as good as their indexing, and hand searching is the most thorough and accurate search method.

AMED

AMED is the Allied and Complementary Medicine database. It is produced by the British Library Health Care Information Service. It contains bibliographic references from 1985 onwards, covering the fields of complementary and allied medicine, in three specific areas: professionals allied to medicine; complementary medicine and palliative care. The scope and coverage of the database is predominantly European, with English as the most common language, and includes references to articles in some 590 relevant journals as well as accessing relevant topics in a more general spread of journals. The following OT journals are included in AMED's journal list:

- *American Journal of Occupational Therapy*
- *Australian Occupational Therapy Journal*
- *British Journal of Occupational Therapy*
- *Canadian Journal of Occupational Therapy*
- *International Journal of Therapy and Rehabilitation*
- *Journal of Occupational Science – Australia*
- *Occupational Therapy in Health Care*
- *Occupational Therapy in Mental Health*
- *Occupational Therapy International*
- *Occupational Therapy Now*
- *OTJR: Occupation, Participation and Health*
- *OT Practice*
- *Physical and Occupational Therapy in Geriatrics*
- *Physical and Occupational Therapy in Pediatrics*
- *Scandinavian Journal of Occupational Therapy*
- *South African Journal of Occupational Therapy*

The thesaurus uses a modified form of the MeSH (medical subject headings) headings. AMED is available via the internet or on CD-ROM, and in both Ovid and SilverPlatter format. Access to AMED is via subscription, although National Health Service (NHS) professionals in England and Wales have free access to AMED through NHSnet. More details are also available from the website (www.bl.uk/collections/health/amed.html).

Although AMED is an extremely useful resource for the evidence-based occupational therapist, it does appear to be somewhat 'selective' in its indexing. Articles that should be identified in a search are sometimes missed when searching AMED. All items included in AMED are available from the British Library Document Supply Centre.

ASSIA

ASSIA is the Applied Social Sciences Index and Abstracts. ASSIA was established in 1987 and is designed to serve the information needs of the caring professions, covering a wide range of topic areas relevant to health and social care. The core areas of coverage in ASSIA are: social problems, healthcare, social services and sociological and psychological issues. Over 500 English-language journals are included, and although the majority of journals are based in the UK or USA, journals from across the English-speaking world are also included. OT-specific journals include:

- *American Journal of Occupational Therapy*
- *Australian Occupational Therapy Journal*
- *British Journal of Occupational Therapy*
- *Occupational Therapy International*
- *Scandinavian Journal of Occupational Therapy*

A useful guide to ASSIA is available from the website (www.csa.com/factsheets/assia-set-c.php).

CINAHL

CINAHL is the Cumulated Index to Nursing and Allied Health Literature. It is produced by CINAHL Information Systems in California. As its name suggests, it provides a database for nursing and allied literature. Like MEDLINE, CINAHL has a somewhat US bias. The majority of journals included in CINAHL have a nursing focus. However, some 43 therapy-related journals are included and of these 14 are specific to OT. The OT-specific journals include:

- *American Journal of Occupational Therapy*
- *Australian Occupational Therapy Journal*
- *British Journal of Occupational Therapy*
- *Canadian Journal of Occupational Therapy*
- *Journal of Occupational Science – Australia*
- *New Zealand Journal of Occupational Therapy*
- *Occupational Therapy in Health Care*
- *Occupational Therapy in Mental Health*
- *Occupational Therapy International*
- *Occupational Therapy Journal of Research*
- *OT Practice*
- *Physical and Occupational Therapy in Geriatrics*
- *Physical and Occupational Therapy in Pediatrics*
- *Scandinavian Journal of Occupational Therapy*

Other journals included in CINAHL, which might be of interest, include:

- *Activities, Adaptation and Aging*
- *Assistive Technology*
- *Therapy Weekly*
- *WORK: A Journal of Prevention, Assessment and Rehabilitation*

CINAHL uses a modified MeSH thesaurus. More details can be found at the CINAHL website (http://www.cinahl.com/).

The Cochrane Library

The Cochrane Library is an electronic library 'designed to provide the evidence needed for healthcare decision making' (Gray 2001, p. 222). The Cochrane Library is published by John Wiley on behalf of the Cochrane Collaboration. The Cochrane Collaboration is an international organization that prepares systematic reviews on the effects and effectiveness of healthcare interventions. The Cochrane Library is a unique resource, providing access to these systematic reviews, as well as a number of other resources. The Cochrane Library is available online and on CD-ROM and is updated quarterly. As well as the Cochrane Database of Systematic reviews it includes a number of other databases including:

▪ Database of Abstracts of Reviews of Effectiveness (DARE) (see below)
▪ Cochrane Central Register of Controlled Trials
▪ Health Technology Assessment Database
▪ NHS Economic Evaluation Database

The Cochrane Library is freely available in England via the National Electronic Library for Health (www.nelh.nhs.uk/cochrane.asp).

Databases such as AMED and MEDLINE include articles because they have been published in the journals that the database includes in its listing. The merits of the article are based on the fact that the journal chose to publish it and that the database chose to include that journal in its listings. No attempt is made to exclude articles on the basis of their research type or because they are not research-based. The Cochrane Library is different. The Cochrane Library contains only research-based information. In fact, all of the information in the Cochrane Library is based on randomized controlled trials (RCTs) and controlled clinical trials (CCTs), which explains why the Cochrane Library might seem of limited value in the search for OT-relevant literature. This is not the case as OT literature is being included in the Controlled Trials Register and occupational therapists are involved with Systematic Review groups.

The Cochrane Database of Systematic Reviews

Systematic reviews were discussed in detail in Chapter 4. Throughout the world groups of researchers work together in Cochrane Collaboration Groups to collate and review the research evidence for specific healthcare interventions. The output from these groups, in the form of review protocols and completed reviews, is made available to a wider audience through the Cochrane Database of Systematic Reviews. Review groups of interest to occupational therapists include:

▪ Occupational Therapy for Parkinson's Disease
▪ Occupational Therapy for Rheumatoid Arthritis
▪ Occupational Therapy for Multiple Sclerosis
▪ Occupational Therapy for Patients with Problems in Activities of Daily Living after Stroke

▦ Occupational Therapy and Physiotherapy for Developmental Coordination Disorder
▦ Cognitive Rehabilitation for People with Schizophrenia and Related Conditions
▦ Work Conditioning, Work Hardening and Functional Restoration for Workers with Back and Neck Pain
▦ Fall Prevention in the Elderly
▦ Hip Fracture: In-patient Rehabilitation
▦ Hospital at Home
▦ Life Skills Programmes for Schizophrenia
▦ Reality Orientation for Dementia
▦ Reminiscence Therapy for Dementia

The Cochrane Collaboration now has a Rehabilitation and Related Therapies Field, which is coordinated through the University of Maastricht and can be contacted via email (ra.deBie@epid.unimaas.nl) or via the website (http://www.cebp.nl).

The Cochrane Controlled Trials Register

The aim of the Cochrane Controlled Trials Register is to index all randomized controlled trials and controlled clinical trials, thus providing a comprehensive database for evidence-based practice. Trials are identified by volunteers hand-searching relevant journals. OT-specific journals are now being hand-searched and included on the Register. This is a painstaking process. However, the Cochrane Controlled Trials Register does now include information pertinent to occupational therapists.

A number of very useful training resources and User Guides are available on the Cochrane Library site, and the reader is strongly recommended to access these to help navigate a path to the most appropriate evidence within the Cochrane Library.

DARE

The Database of Abstracts of Reviews of Effectiveness (DARE) is produced by the NHS Centre for Reviews and Dissemination (CRD; see below). DARE provides a record of good-quality research-based reviews of the effectiveness of health and social care interventions, management and organization. The staff at NHS CRD evaluate the reviews against quality criteria and provide abstracts of reviews that meet the quality standards. This information can, therefore, be regarded as 'kite-marked' for research quality. DARE also includes records of other useful reviews that do not meet the quality standards. DARE can be viewed as a source of over-views of high-quality reviews of evidence. However, because of its quantitative focus, DARE may be of limited value for many occupational therapists.

DARE is available online at the website (www.york.ac.uk/inst/crd/crddatabases.htm). It is also available via:

- The Cochrane Library.
- TRIP (Turning Evidence into Practice) – DARE is one of the databases searched when using the TRIP database (www.tripdatabase.com/index.html).
- SUMSearch (www.sumsearch.uthscsa.edu) – this is a meta-search engine that searches multiple internet sites. As well as searching DARE, SUMSearch also identifies relevant documents from the National Library of Medicine (NLM: www.nlm.nih.gov) and the National Guideline Clearinghouse (NGC: www.guidelines.gov).

EMBASE

EMBASE is seen by many people as the European version of MEDLINE. It is produced in the Netherlands by Elsevier Science. As well as having a more European focus it tends to focus on the more pharmacological aspects of medicine. Section 19, Physical Medicine and Rehabilitation, may be of use to occupational therapists. EMBASE is available online by subscription.

MEDLINE

MEDLINE is the world's largest and most popular medical database. It is produced by the US National Library of Medicine (NLM). The printed version of the database (Index Medicus) was started in the 1870s by John Shaw Billings. The database was computerized in 1966 and became known as MEDLINE. Now it is also available via the internet as PubMed (see below). The journals included in MEDLINE are all peer reviewed, and as the name suggests, the focus is on medical rather than related journals. Of the 5000 plus journals included in MEDLINE only four are OT journals, namely:

- *American Journal of Occupational Therapy*
- *Occupational Therapy International*
- *Physical and Occupational Therapy in Pediatrics*
- *Scandinavian Journal of Occupational Therapy*

However, other relevant journals included are:

- *Alternative Therapies in Health and Medicine*
- *American Journal of Physical Medicine and Rehabilitation*
- *International Journal of Rehabilitation Research*

MEDLINE is available online and on CD-ROM, and because of its popularity is available in most medical libraries. Whilst MEDLINE might not be the first database to choose for evidence-based OT, it will give access to some OT literature and to a reasonable range of background medical literature. The thesaurus uses the MeSH system.

National Research Register

The National Research Register (NRR) is a register of ongoing and recently completed research projects funded by, or of interest to, the NHS. It contains information on over 28 000 research projects, as well as information from the UK's Medical Research Council's (MRC) Clinical Trials Register, and details of systematic reviews currently in progress from the NHS CRD, as well as abstracts of Cochrane Reviews. It is the most comprehensive register of current NHS research. As such it has great value as a source of information on unpublished research and as a way of accessing the full scope of NHS research. The Register uses the MeSH thesaurus as an indexing tool. The NRR can be accessed for free, via the internet, from the NRR website (www.nrr.nhs.uk).

OT BibSys/OT Search

OT BibSys/OT Search is a database covering both the OT literature and related topic areas, such as rehabilitation, education, psychiatry, psychology and healthcare delivery. It provides bibliographic information and abstracts for the material listed. The database is run by the American Occupational Therapy Association (AOTA) and the American Occupational Therapy Foundation (AOTF) (see below). All of the material listed in OT BibSys/OT Search is held at the Wilma L. West Library (part of AOTF) and inter-library loan or photocopies can be requested from the Library. The aim of the database is to bring together OT literature into one database, so the non-OT-specific literature is limited to such literature written by occupational therapists or of direct interest to them. The thesaurus for OT BibSys/OT Search is based on MeSH.

OT BibSys/OT Search is not a free service. There are four subscription categories:

- individual member (member of AOTA)
- individual student member
- individual non-member
- institution

The individual non-member rate is currently US$200 per year. Access to the database is via the OT BibSys website (http://www.aotf.org/otsearch.html).

OTDBASE

OTDBASE is a database of OT journal literature. It was developed by a Canadian occupational therapist, Marilyn Ernest-Conibear. The database contains abstracts from 25 OT journals and is indexed using 18 OT subject areas, giving some 240 topic areas, with new topic areas being added as the profession develops. Entries are cross-referenced wherever possible to make searching as comprehensive and as simple as possible. The database is updated monthly. The database can only be accessed online by subscription to OTDBASE. Some national OT associations are subscribers as are some universities; individual subscribers can subscribe by the month. A useful option for non-subscribers is the OTDBASE open house, which happens twice a year for about a month and gives anyone an opportunity to explore OTDBASE and to assess its value as a potential evidence-based occupational therapy resource.

OTDBASE claims to be fast and easy to use. All entries are cross-referenced. Having chosen *one* key term from the main index (e.g. mental health), you are then given a further list of key terms to choose from (e.g. activity, depression); you will then be given a list of all the relevant references in the OTDBASE indexed journals. The beauty of this service is its simplicity. However, this is also its limitation, as the *index* supplies the search terms, not the searcher. The other limitation of OTDBASE is that it is a database exclusively of OT literature. Thus, it will not index articles written by occupational therapists, or about OT, but published in non-OT journals. The citations include bibliographic information and the article abstract. OTDBASE claims to be easier to use, and more comprehensive (in terms of journal information) than OT BibSys. However, OT BibSys includes conference proceedings and other information, which OTDBASE does not. OTDBASE can be accessed via the website (www.otdbase.org).

OTseeker

A detailed overview of this useful database is given in Chapter 6. OTseeker is a database of systematic reviews and RCTs that are of relevance to occupational therapists. It can be accessed via the website (www.otseeker.com).

PEDro

The Physiotherapy Evidence Database (PEDro) was the precursor to OTseeker and contains bibliographic details and abstracts of RCTs, systematic reviews and evidence-based clinical practice guidelines in physiotherapy. Like OTseeker, the majority of the RCTs included in the database have been quality rated. It can be accessed via the website (www.pedro.fhs.usyd.edu.au).

Websites

This section does not claim to include an exhaustive list of relevant sites. Rather, it aims to give an overview of websites that the author has found particularly useful or noteworthy. Other websites are included within entries in other more relevant sections (e.g. COT website, AOTA website).

▪ ▪

Activity

As a way of developing your own list of favourite web-based evidence-based OT resources, it might be useful to type 'evidence based practice' into a search engine, such as Google, and review the range of resources available.

▪ ▪

CASP: the Critical Skills Appraisal Programme (www.phru.nhs.uk/casp/casp.htm)

CASP's aim is to help health service professionals develop skills in the critical appraisal of evidence about effectiveness and to promote the delivery of evidence-based healthcare. CASP runs half-day workshops on the key skills of finding and making sense of evidence to support healthcare decisions. CASP also runs training-the-trainer workshops, to help people develop the skills of teaching critical appraisal skills. CASP has also developed an open learning resource and an interactive CD-ROM on evidence-based healthcare. The CASP website has links to a variety of useful learning resources.

Centre for Evidence-based Medicine (www.cebm.net)

The Centre for Evidence-based Medicine was opened in March 1995. Its remit is:

> to promote the teaching and practice of evidence-based health care throughout the UK . . . to effect the creation of formal graduate education in the conduct of randomised controlled trials and systematic reviews in the University of Oxford

Although its focus is predominantly medical, the CEBM is a valuable resource for the evidence-based occupational therapist. The CEBM website is well worth a visit, as it contains teaching resources as well as useful links to other evidence-based websites.

Centre for Evidence-based Mental Health (www.cebmh.com)

This website provides access to a range of evidence and resources of particular interest to those working with people experiencing mental health problems. This is a useful resource for all mental health practitioners. It also has excellent links to other evidence-based mental health sites and aims to give users access to high-quality evidence in *less than three clicks*, by using key words to allow access to evidence-based information on the internet.

EBOT Portal (www.otevidence.info)

A detailed overview of this useful database is given in Chapter 6.

Google Scholar (scholar.google.com)

Google Scholar provides a free search engine that provides access to scholarly literature across the internet. Google Scholar is easy to search. However, it does not have access to journals from all scholarly publishers and so any search may miss key papers.

Joanna Briggs Institute (www.joannabriggs.edu.au/about/home.php)

The Joanna Briggs Institute is an international Research and Development Unit of the Royal Adelaide Hospital. The Institute was set up because of a recognized need for a collaborative approach to the evaluation of evidence derived from a diverse range of sources, including experience, expertise and all forms of rigorous research, and the translation, transfer and utilization of the 'best available' evidence into healthcare practice. The website has both public and members-only content, which provides a range of resources and evidence for the evidence-based occupational therapist. The Institute is particularly involved in the use of qualitative research within the evidence-based context.

NARIC: the National Rehabilitation Information Center (www.naric.com)

This US resource and website gives access to various NARIC databases. These include listings of current research covered by the National Institute of Disability and Rehabilitation Research (NIDRR) programme, current and historical (pre-1993) rehabilitation literature and the NARIC Knowledgebase (an information resource). The databases can be searched or browsed, and seem to hold a wide range of potentially useful information.

New Zealand Guidelines Group (NZGG) (www.nzgg.org.nz)

The New Zealand Guidelines Group, like SIGN (see below), aims to ensure that healthcare delivery is effective and based on an evidence-based approach, through the development of guidelines for practice. As well as giving access to a variety of guidelines, the site also contains much valuable information on the development and utilization of guidelines for practice.

NHS Centre for Reviews and Dissemination (www.york.ac.uk/inst/crd)

The NHS Centre for Reviews and Dissemination (CRD) is commissioned by the NHS R&D Directorate to produce and disseminate reviews concerning the effectiveness and cost-effectiveness of healthcare interventions. The aim of CRD is to identify and review the results of good-quality health research and to disseminate actively the findings to key decision-makers in the NHS and to consumers of healthcare services. In this way healthcare professionals and managers can ensure their practice reflects the best available research evidence. The reviews cover the effectiveness of care for particular conditions; the effectiveness of health technologies; and evidence about efficient methods of organizing and delivering particular types of healthcare. The reviews are collected into a database of structured abstracts of good-quality systematic reviews (DARE), which comment on the methodological features of published reviews and summarize the conclusions of the author(s) and any implications for health practice. The abstracts represent the end product of a detailed sifting and quality appraisal process.

OT CATs (www.otcats.com)

CATs are *critically appraised topics* (and were discussed in more detail in Chapter 8). This site contains CATs on OT interventions and, as such, provides a useful resource for the evidence-based occupational therapist.

OTdirect (www.otdirect.co.uk)

OT*direct* is an independent site for occupational therapists, OT assistants and OT students, produced by occupational therapists in their spare time. It aims to provide not only links to useful resources on the web, but also study notes, practice updates and training listings.

PubMed (www.ncbi.nlm.nih.gov/entrez/query.fcgi)

PubMed is MEDLINE on the web. It allows *free* access to the MEDLINE database. This means that anyone can search MEDLINE via the internet. However, PubMed can only offer simple searching using one or two key words, and the citations provided do not include the article abstracts. PubMed can, however, be a useful place to begin a search.

The NLM, who produce PubMed, have also recently launched MedlinePlus (medlineplus.gov/), which aims to provide an easy-to-understand resource for the public. It includes MEDLINE as well as links to self-help groups and information on clinical trials. Apart from links to numerous sources, it also has preformatted MEDLINE searches on a number of popular topics.

Research in Practice for Adults (www.ripfa.org.uk)

This is a useful evidence-based OT resource, particularly for occupational thera-pists working in a social care context, with links to a range of evidence sources including research and policy. The website also has links to SCIE (the Social Care Institute for Excellence).

School of Health and Related Research (ScHARR) at Sheffield University (www.shef.ac.uk/scharr/ir/netting/)

ScHARR is a multidisciplinary research centre that covers medical, allied and social science perspectives on healthcare. It is part of the Trent Institute of Health Services Research. ScHARR produces a number of evidence-based resources. The website consists of an A–Z guide and introduction to evidence-based practice on the internet. The site also has links to evidence-based practice tutorials and a range of evidence-based practice-related resources worldwide.

Scottish Intercollegiate Guidelines Network (SIGN) (www.sign.ac.uk)

The Scottish Intercollegiate Guidelines Network (SIGN) was formed in 1993. Its objective is to improve the quality of healthcare for patients in Scotland by reduc-ing variation in practice and outcome, through the development and dissemina-tion of national clinical guidelines containing recommendations for effective practice based on current evidence. SIGN has a programme of 113 evidence-based clinical guidelines – published, in development or under review – covering a wide range of topics. Many of the SIGN guidelines relate to the NHS priority areas of cancer, cardiovascular disease and mental health. (See also NZGG above.)

Teaching and Learning Resources for Evidence Based Practice (www.mdx.ac.uk/www/rctsh/ebp/main.htm)

This site contains a range of resources and teaching materials for evidence-based practice (EBP), designed for an audience of nurses and professionals allied to medicine (PAMs). Amongst the materials on the site are outlines for introductory courses on EBP and a wealth of other teaching materials. This is an excellent place to start if you have to devise a session on EBP.

Email discussion groups

Email discussion groups allow groups of people with similar areas of interest to discuss ideas, issues, etc. via the internet. One person poses a question or makes a comment, and other list members reply. There are a number of discussion groups, a few of which are described briefly below.

Critical Appraisal Skills Discussion List
(email: critical-appraisal-skills@mailbase.ac.uk)

This relatively new UK-based list is linked to the CASP International network. The aim of the list is to provide a forum for the exchange of information, ideas and experience about finding, critically appraising and using evidence as part of healthcare delivery. The list is both multiprofessional and international in its membership. To join, send the message 'join critical-appraisal-skills *your name*' to mailbase@mailbase.ac.uk.

Evidence-based Health Discussion List
(email: evidence-based-medicine@mailbase.ac.uk)

This UK-based discussion group is aimed at practitioners and teachers in all healthcare-related areas. The main goal of the group is to assist the implementation of evidence-based healthcare. The list is also used to debate and discuss issues relevant to evidence-based practice, to announce meetings and courses, and to seek information and answers to questions. To join, send the message 'join evidence-based-health *your name*' to mailbase@mailbase.ac.uk.

Occup-ther (email: occup-ther@ac.dal.ca)

This Canadian-based OT list is administered by Barbara O'Shea at Dalhousie University. The list is open to qualified occupational therapists only. The list has members throughout the world, although the majority of discussions tend to have a North American slant. However, access to several hundred occupational therapists around the world can provide useful information and ideas about interventions and evidence in OT. To join, send the message 'subscribe occup-ther *your name*' to occup-ther-request@ac.dal.ca.

Occupational-therapy (email: occupational-therapy@mailbase.ac.uk)

This is a UK-based OT discussion list. There tends to be considerable overlap between occup-ther and occupational-therapy. UK occupational therapists seem to subscribe, and send the same messages, to both lists, although non-UK-based occupational therapists tend to subscribe to occup-ther. To join, send the message 'join occupational-therapy *your name*' to mailbase@mailbase.ac.uk.

Further reading

Key texts

Bury, T. & Mead, J. (1998) *Evidence-Based Healthcare.* Oxford: Butterworth-Heinemann.
This book is aimed at therapists in general. It provides an overview of evidence-based practice and uses case examples to illustrate ideas. It includes some information on finding and appraising evidence. However, its main focus is on implementing change through an evidence-based approach. Its approach is more global than practical. It might be a useful resource for therapy managers and people involved in establishing evidence-based policy at a local level.

Gray, J.A.M. (2001) *Evidence-Based Healthcare,* 2nd edn. Edinburgh: Churchill Livingstone.
This book deals with evidence-based practice from the perspective of policy and management. Gray gives a general introduction to finding and appraising evidence. However, the main focus of the book is on using evidence to develop healthcare policy and management at local levels and beyond. This is a book for evidence-based managers rather than for evidence-based practitioners.

Greenhalgh, T. (2006) *How to Read a Paper,* 3rd edn. Oxford: Blackwell Publishing.
This book provides a very clear and readable introduction to evidence-based medicine. It includes chapters on finding and appraising a variety of types of published evidence. It is a useful introduction, but the reader must remember that it is written from a *medical* perspective.

Greyson, L. (1997) *Evidence-Based Medicine: an Overview and Guide to the Literature.* London: The British Library.
Whilst this book contains some discussion of the nature of evidence-based medicine, its main focus is to provide an overview of the source of literature and other evidence pertinent to an evidence-based approach. As well as reviewing sources of evidence this book also outlines literature relevant to getting the evidence into practice. Although this book has a rather medical focus, it does provide a useful resource for the evidence-based practitioner.

Langhorne, P. & Dennis, M. (1998) *Stroke Units: an Evidence Based Approach.* London: BMJ Publishing Group.
Using the Cochrane Stroke Unit Collaboration systematic review as a basis, this book gives an overview of the role of inpatient stroke units in the care and management of stroke patients. It reviews the evidence for the effectiveness of stroke unit care. The book reviews the economics of stroke units and the implications of using the evidence to plan services for stroke patients. This concise volume provides excellent background both to stroke care and to the use of evidence to underpin rehabilitation service delivery.

Li Wan Po, A. (1998) *Dictionary of Evidence-Based Medicine.* Abingdon: Radcliffe Medical Press.
An excellent source of definitions of the common terms of evidence-based practice, especially the technical language of biostatistics, epidemiology and health economics. The author has included a number of references for the enthusiastic reader to follow up discussion of some of the terms and concepts.

Pereira-Maxwell, F. (1998) *A–Z of Medical Statistics: a Companion for Critical Appraisal.* London: Arnold.
This useful little book uses a dictionary format to provide the reader with a succinct overview of medical statistics. It is not intended to be a comprehensive medical statistics textbook. Rather, it provides the evidence-based practitioner with a collection of simple explanations of the key statistical terms and concepts frequently encountered when attempting to read and critically appraise research evidence.

Strauss, S.E., Richardson, W.S., Glasziou, P., & Haynes, R.B. (2005) *Evidence-Based Medicine: How to Practice and Teach EBM,* 3rd edn. Edinburgh: Churchill Livingstone.
This pocket-sized book is designed to be an instant resource for evidence-based medicine. It is aimed at doctors and its focus is totally medical. However, it provides useful, basic information about using and teaching evidence-based practice.

Evidence-based journals and other books and publications

Bandolier

Bandolier is a monthly newsletter on evidence-based healthcare produced by Oxford Anglia NHS Region R&D Directorate. Its format is bullet points of information about evidence-based medicine, hence the name *Bandolier*. It is available in printed form or via the internet. Internet access is free, although the most up-to-date version is not usually available. The subscription for the print version is currently £36 a year. It is available from: Pain Relief Clinic, The Churchill Hospital, Headington, Oxford, OX3 7LJ
or via the website (http://www.jr2.ox.ac.uk/Bandolier).
This site also has good links to other related and evidence-based sites.

Effective Health Care bulletins

The *Effective Health Care* bulletins, which are produced by the NHS Centre for Reviews and Dissemination, are available on the world wide web at
www.york.ac.uk/inst/crd/ehcb.htm
They are also available bimonthly in printed form. These bulletins are designed to help healthcare decision-makers, by examining the effectiveness of various healthcare interventions. The information in each bulletin is based on systematic reviews and a synthesis of the research on clinical effectiveness, cost-effectiveness and acceptability of the particular healthcare intervention being discussed. Each bulletin is subjected to rigorous peer review. *Effective Health Care* bulletins should be viewed as excellent sources of information on clinical effectiveness of interventions for the evidence-based occupational therapist.

Journals

Australian Occupational Therapy Journal [regularly contains at least four critically appraised papers]
Clinical Evidence
Evidence-based Child Health
Evidence-based Health Policy and Management
Evidence-based Medicine
Evidence-based Mental Health
Evidence-based Nursing
Focus on Alternative and Complementary Therapies
Physical Therapy [includes a section 'Evidence in Practice']

Books

Bailey, D.M. (1997) *Research for the Health Professional,* 2nd edn. Philadelphia: FA Davis Co.

Chalmers, I. & Altman, D.G. (eds) (1995) *Systematic Reviews.* London: BMJ Publishing Group.

Crombie, I.K. (1996) *Pocket Guide to Critical Appraisal*. London: BMJ Publishing Group.

Crump, B. & Drummond, M.F. (1993) *Evaluating Clinical Evidence: a Handbook for Managers*. London: Longman.

DePoy, E. & Gitlin, L.N. (1994) *Introduction to Research*. St Louis: Mosby.

Dixon, R.A., Munro, J.F. & Silcocks, P.B. (1997) *The Evidence Based Medicine Workbook*. Oxford: Butterworth-Heinemann.

Dunning, M., Abi-Aad, G., Gilbert, D., Gillam, S. & Livett, H. (1998) *Turning Evidence into Everyday Practice*. London: King's Fund.

Entwistle, V., Watts, I.S. & Herring, J.E. (1997) *Information About Health Care Effectiveness*. London: King's Fund.

Grbich, C. (1999) *Qualitative Research in Health*. London: Sage.

Hope, T. (1997) *Evidence-Based Patient Choice*. London: King's Fund.

Lockett, T. (1997) *Evidence-Based and Cost-Effective Medicine for the Uninitiated*. London: Radcliffe Medical Press

McQuay, H. & Moore, A. (1998) *An Evidence-Based Resource for Pain Relief*. Oxford: Oxford University Press.

Munro, B.H. & Page, E.B. (1993) *Statistical Methods for Health Care Research*. Philadelphia: J.B. Lippincott Co.

Peckham, M. & Smith, R. (eds) (1996) *Scientific Basis of Health Care*. London: BMJ Publishing Group.

Robson, C. (1993) *Real World Research*. Oxford: Blackwell.

Sinclair, A. & Dickinson, E. (1998) *Effective Practice in Rehabilitation*. London: King's Fund.

Useful addresses and other miscellaneous resources

AOTA/AOTF

The American Occupational Therapy Association (AOTA)
The American Occupational Therapy Foundation (AOTF)

4720 Montgomery Lane, PO Box 31220, Bethesda, MD 20824-1220, USA
☎ 301-652-2682
Fax: 301-652-7711
Email: aota@aota.org
        aotf@aotf.org
Website: http://www.aota.org
        http://www.aotf.org

AOTA is the professional society for occupational therapists in the USA, representing the interests of OT and its US practitioners. It produces a number of publications including: *American Journal of Occupational Therapy, OT Practice* and *OT Week*.

AOTF is a charitable, scientific, educational and literary organization that aims to expand and refine the body of knowledge of OT and promote the understanding of the value of occupation. AOTF supports scholarship and research into OT in the USA. It acts as a resource base for OT, through its own library, the Wilma L. West Library, and OT BibSys (see above). AOTF publishes the *Occupational Therapy Journal of Research*.

The AOTF website contains access to a database of assessments related to OT, a database of rehabilitation organizations in the USA, a listing of online databases relevant to rehabilitation and OT, and links to useful OT and non-OT websites.

CAOT

Canadian Association of Occupational Therapists (CAOT)

CTTC, Suite 3400, 1125 Colonel By Drive, Ottawa, Ontario, Canada, K1S 5R1
☎ (613) 523-2268
Fax: (613) 523-2552
Website: http://www.caot.ca

CAOT is the professional association for occupational therapists in Canada. It publishes the following journals: *Canadian Journal of Occupational Therapy* and *Occupational Therapy Now*. It has also been instrumental in the formulation of client-centred practice within OT.

The College of Occupational Therapists (COT)

106–114 Borough High St, Southwark, London, SE1 1LB
☎ 020 7357 6480
Fax: 020 7250 2299
Website: http:/www.cot.co.uk

The College of Occupational Therapists is the professional body for occupational therapists in the UK. Its Library and Information Service, which is available to members, can be accessed by telephone, fax, written query, email or visited in person. The Library holds a collection of OT journals as well as a thesis and dissertation collection. There are reference facilities including CINAHL and AMED. The Library produces Current Awareness Bulletins and factsheets, can provide photocopies of reference material, and lend dissertations and theses.

The address of the Library is the same as COT (above)
☎ 020 7450 2316
Fax: 020 7450 2299

University of Oxford Department of Continuing Education

1 Wellington Square, Oxford, OX1 2JA
☎ 01865 280347
Fax: 01865 270386
Website: www.conted.ox.ac.uk

The University of Oxford's Centre for Continuing Professional Development runs the Oxford Master's Programme in Evidence-Based Health Care. The Programme is modular and part-time. It consists of three, related, courses: Postgraduate Certificate; Postgraduate Diploma; and MSc. The Programme is aimed at professionals working in any area of healthcare. The Centre also runs a series of short courses on all aspects of evidence-based practice.

Glossary

AMED: Allied and Complementary Medicine database; a useful source of references of specific relevance to the evidence-based occupational therapist. *See* Chapters 2 & 10.

ASSIA (Applied Social Science Index of Abstracts): a key source for social science references, with good coverage of applied social care topics. *See* Chapters 2 & 10.

Bandolier: a monthly newsletter that focuses on evidence-based practice and gives brief overviews of relevant issues. *See* Chapter 10.

Bias: the systematic deviation of results from the true value of the results. There are two main sources of bias in intervention research: poor sampling, which will lead to non-representative groups of participants being used in a study; and problems with the process of the study or the measurement tools used in the study.

Blind: describing a trial or other study in which researchers and/or the participants are unaware of which experimental group the participant is in, thereby ensuring that the researcher and/or the participant are not influenced by knowing that they are in the experimental or the control group. *Single blind* studies are studies in which the participants are unaware of which intervention they are receiving. *Double blind* studies are studies where both the participants and the health professionals administering the interventions are unaware of whether the participant is part of the intervention or the control group.

Boolean operators: words such as AND, OR and NOT that are used to refine search terms when carrying out literature searches. *See* Chapter 2.

CAP (critically appraised paper): a research paper for which someone has already done the hard work of appraisal. A CAP usually consists of an overview of the research study and a commentary. The commentary usually includes both a review of the research methodology and rigour of the research paper and comments on the value of the study to the evidence-based practitioner. Occupational therapy CAPs are now a regular feature in the *Australian Occupational Therapy Journal*.

CASP (Critical Appraisal Skills Programme): an organization that runs workshops to help practitioners develop their critical appraisal skills. It also produces distance learning packs and a CD-ROM to help practitioners refine their evidence-based skills. *See* Chapter 10.

CAT (critically appraised topic): effectively a small-scale systematic review, in which the reviewer has developed a question, looked for relevant evidence, appraised the evidence and presented the essential findings. *See* 'OT CATs' in Chapter 10.

CCT *see* **controlled clinical trial**.

CI *see* **confidence interval**.

CINAHL (Cumulative Index of Nursing and Allied Health Literature): a database of predominantly nursing literature, with some rehabilitation and allied health literature. *See* Chapters 2 & 10.

Clinical effectiveness (*or* effectiveness): the extent to which a particular intervention/procedure/service improves the outcome for the clients. The extent to which the intervention achieves its intended purpose for a broad range of clients/patients receiving the outcome in practice. *Compare* **efficacy**, which refers to the ideal or restricted parameters of a randomized controlled trial.

Clinical governance: the philosophy and framework through which organizations in the UK's National Health Service (NHS) are accountable for continually assessing and improving the quality of the services they provide.

Clinical guidelines: systematically developed statements that aim to help practitioners and clients make rational decisions about the most appropriate healthcare for specific problems.

Clinical significance: is seen in terms of the size of a treatment effect, expressed in terms of *odds ratios* and *numbers needed to treat*. Deciding how large the treatment effect should be before an intervention is seen as clinically significant is a matter of practitioner judgment. Studies may be *statistically significant* without being clinically significant.

Cochrane Collaboration: a collaborative network focusing on carrying out, and making accessible, systematic reviews of *randomized controlled trials* of healthcare. The collaboration began with the establishment of the UK Cochrane Centre but the collaboration is now international with a number of national centres coordinating the work of review groups and networks. The main output of the collaboration is the *Cochrane Library*.

Cochrane Library: a quarterly publication (on disk/CD-ROM and via the internet) produced by the *Cochrane Collaboration*. It consists of a number of separate databases: the Cochrane Database of Systematic Reviews; Database of Abstracts of Reviews of Effectiveness (DARE) (see below); Cochrane Central Register of

Controlled Trials; Health Technology Assessment Database; and the NHS Economic Evaluation Database. *See* Chapter 10.

Confidence interval (CI): the range of values within which the 'true' result can be found, with a given level of confidence. Commonly accepted confidence intervals are 95% or 99%. This means that the true result lies somewhere within the range in 95% (or 99%) of cases. *See* Chapter 3.

Confirmability: the strategies used by a qualitative researcher to limit bias within her or his research. *See* Chapter 5.

Controlled clinical trial (CCT): a trial in which interventions are compared but it is not possible (for practical or ethical reasons) to randomly *(see randomization)* allocate the participants to the various study groups, as in a *randomized controlled trial*. *See* Chapter 3.

Controls (*or* control group): the participants in a randomized controlled trial *(see below)* who provide the comparison group. They receive the standard intervention (or a *placebo*, or no intervention) so that their outcomes can be compared with those of the experimental group in order to assess the *efficacy* of the intervention under trial.

Credibility: used to assess the rigour of qualitative research. It refers to whether the research is giving a true picture of the phenomenon being studied. A good test of credibility is whether the descriptions and interpretations of the phenomenon being researched are recognizable to people outside the research setting. *See* Chapter 5.

Critical appraisal: the process of reviewing, assessing and interpreting evidence by systematically considering its rigour, results and relevance to your own area of practice. *See also* **CASP**.

DARE (Database of Reviews of Effectiveness): a database produced by the NHS Centre for Reviews and Dissemination (NHS CRD) at York University. It contains quality-assessed systematic reviews and is a valuable source of high-quality evidence for the evidence-based occupational therapist. *See* Chapter 10.

Data extraction: the process, when carrying out a systematic review, of identifying and recording all the relevant information from the various research studies to be included within the review. It is usually carried out systematically using some form of data extraction tool. *See* Chapter 8.

Dependability: a technique for assessing the rigour of a piece of qualitative research. It relates to how consistent the data and findings of the study are. *See* Chapter 5.

Effectiveness *see* **clinical effectiveness**.

Efficacy: the extent to which an intervention improves the outcome for patients under ideal circumstances. *Compare* **clinical effectiveness**.

Ethnography: a method of qualitative research. The main focus of ethnographic studies is the exploration of cultures. *See* Chapter 5.

Experimental group (*or* experimental condition): the group of participants in a randomized controlled trial who receive the intervention. If the outcome for this group is better compared with the *control group*, the trial can be seen as providing evidence for the *efficacy* of the intervention.

Free text searching: when natural (or everyday) language and terms are used as the search terms in a literature search.

Generalizability: a term used especially within quantitative research to indicate how well the results of one study can be applied to a more general population.

Gold standard: what is generally regarded as the best available evidence, method or measure. In evidence-based medicine *randomized controlled trials* are seen as the gold standard for evidence, against which all other research is compared and found wanting.

Heterogeneity: differences in results or participant groups. Heterogeneity is often assessed in *systematic reviews* and *meta-analyses*, when the results for the various studies appear to be markedly different. If there is evidence of heterogeneity a single summary of the individual results within a review should not be given. Systematic reviews often include tests of heterogeneity; however, these tests are not very powerful and can be confusing. Individual judgment and appraisal is probably the best assessment of heterogeneity. *Compare* **homogeneity**.

Homogeneity: a measure of the similarity of a group of research participants or results. Studies are said to be homogeneous if the spread of their results is less than would be expected as chance variations. Homogeneous subject (or participant) groups are groups of people who are similar along the defined parameters of the study (e.g. age, gender, social class, diagnosis, length of intervention). *Compare* **heterogeneity**.

Hypothesis: a testable statement, usually stating a cause and effect, that is the basis of experimental research, including *randomized controlled trials*.

Mean: the average value for a particular group of data. It is calculated by adding together all of the measurements (scores) and dividing them by the number of measurements (participants).

Median: the value on a scale, or series of data, that indicates the mid-point in the data set. Half of the observations (scores) are below this number and half are above this number.

MEDLINE: a database of biomedical literature. It is the largest, and most popular, medical database. It is available (by subscription) on CD-ROM. The (free) online version of MEDLINE is *PubMed*. *See* Chapter 10.

MeSH (Medical Subject Heading): the indexing system used by MEDLINE and other health/medical-orientated database systems.

Meta-analysis: a statistical technique, used predominantly in systematic reviews, that summarizes the results of a number of studies into one estimate of the efficacy of an intervention.

NICE (National Institute of Health and Clinical Excellence): an organization set up by the UK Department of Health to promote clinical cost-effectiveness and the production and dissemination of *clinical guidelines*.

Numbers needed to treat (NNT): a measure of the clinical effectiveness of a treatment, and the clinical significance of a systematic review. The NNT is the number of people who would need to be treated with a specific intervention (e.g. admission to a stroke unit) to produce one occurrence of a specific outcome (e.g. prevention of death or dependency).

Odds ratio (OR): a measure of an intervention's clinical effectiveness and clinical significance. It refers to the likelihood of the experimental intervention being effective in comparison with the control intervention. An odds ratio of 1 indicates that there is the same likelihood (odds) of the outcome occurring in both the interaction and the control group. An odds ratio of less than 1 indicates a better outcome in the intervention group, or evidence for the effectiveness of the intervention. An odds ratio of more than 1 indicates better outcomes in the control group, or no evidence for the effectiveness of the intervention. *See* Chapter 4.

OMNI: an internet 'gateway' that gives access to websites of interest to medical practitioners. *See* Chapter 10.

OTBibSys/OTSearch: a database covering both the occupational therapy (OT) literature and related topic areas, such as rehabilitation, education, psychiatry, psychology and healthcare delivery. It provides bibliographic information for the material listed. The database is run by AOTA/AOTF. *See* Chapter 10.

OTDBase: a database of occupational therapy (OT) journal literature. It is available online, by subscription. *See* Chapters 2 & 10.

OTSeeker: a database of systematic reviews and randomized controlled trials that are of relevance to occupational therapists. *See* Chapter 10.

PEDro: the physiotherapy evidence database, similar to *OTSeeker* in format and content. *See* Chapter 10.

PEDro Rating Scale: a ten-item questionnaire designed to assess the quality and rigour of a randomized controlled trial, and frequently used as a quality assessment tool within a systematic review. *See* Chapter 8.

Phenomenology: a qualitative research method. The main focus of phenomenological research is understanding the experience of a particular event (phenomenon) from the perspective of the participant.

Placebo: an inactive treatment often given as part of a randomized controlled trial. The placebo intervention is delivered in a way that makes it appear identical to the experimental intervention, and is a way of eliminating any psychological effects on participants of being in a study.

Probability: the likelihood of any result occurring due to chance, as opposed to the intervention. *See* Chapter 3.

Publication bias: can result if only studies indicating positive or successful findings are published. Although the tendency for journals to publish only 'significant' research is changing, critical appraisers of systematic reviews should be aware that only positive research might be published, or chosen for a review.

PubMed: the (free) online version of *MEDLINE. See* Chapters 2 & 10.

Quality assessment: the process, within a systematic review, of rating the rigour of each of the research papers to be included within the review. It is usually carried out using some form of quality assessment scoring system, such as the PEDro Rating Scale. *See* Chapter 8.

Randomization: the process of allocating participants to various groups within a *randomized controlled trial.* Each participant has the same likelihood of being allocated to the experimental as to the control conditions. Randomization ensures that all participant groups are as similar as possible in terms of key variables (e.g. age, sex, social class). *See* Chapter 3.

Randomized controlled trial (RCT): a study of the effectiveness of an intervention in which the participants have been randomly *(see* **randomization***)* allocated to the various groups (e.g. experimental, control, alternative intervention). *Compare* **controlled clinical trial***. See* Chapter 3.

Reliability: a measure of the rigour of a piece of quantitative research. Reliability implies that the study would give the same results if the measures used were repeated, either by the same researcher or by other researchers.

Review: any summary of the literature on a particular topic. It may include research and non-research literature and, unless it is a *systematic review,* need not have attempted to ensure that all relevant literature is accessed or that the quality of the research is assessed.

Rigour: the circumstance in which a piece of research has been conducted to ensure that any bias is reduced to a minimum, that there is the maximum possible *reliability, validity* or *trustworthiness,* and that the appropriate techniques and strategies have been used to ensure this.

Statistical significance: the result of a statistical test when the associated p value *(see* **probability***)* is found to be below a predetermined cut-off point, conventionally set at $p = 0.05$. Statistical significance is often written as '$p < 0.05$'; however, with modern computer statistical packages it is possible to calculate the exact p value, and this should be stated. *See* Chapter 3.

Systematic review: a review and synthesis of the research literature on a particular topic. A systematic review will attempt to access all published and unpublished literature on the chosen topic. Studies are only included in the review if they meet predetermined criteria of research quality. The findings of the various studies may be combined using meta-analysis, if appropriate. *See* Chapter 4.

Transferability: a way of assessing the rigour of qualitative research. It refers to how well the research achieves 'goodness of fit' with other contexts. It is the task of the appraiser (rather than the researcher) to decide how transferable a piece of research is. *See* Chapter 5.

Triangulation: a strategy for ensuring rigour in qualitative research. It involves collecting data from a number of different sources and utilizing a number of different data collection techniques. *See* Chapter 5.

Trustworthiness: the rigour of a piece of qualitative research. Aspects of trustworthiness in qualitative research include: *credibility, transferability, dependability* and *confirmability*. *See* Chapter 5.

Validity: the rigour of a piece of quantitative research. A study is valid if it does what it set out to do and if the measures used actually measure what they purport to measure.

References

Alderson, P., Green, S. & Higgins, J. (2004) *Cochrane Reviewers' Handbook 4.2.2*. Chichester: John Wiley & Sons.

American Occupational Therapy Association (1996) *Occupational Therapy Practice Guidelines for Adults with Stroke*. Bethesda, MD: American Occupational Therapy Association.

Armitage, P., Berry, G. & Matthews, J.N.S. (2002) *Statistical Methods in Medical Research*, 4th edn. Oxford: Blackwell Science.

Arnold, C., Bain, J., Brown, R. *et al.* (1995) *Moving to Audit: an Education Package for the Professions Allied to Medicine*. Dundee: Centre for Medical Education.

Atherton, C., Barratt, M. & Hodson, R. (2005) *Teamwise: Using Research Evidence: a Practical Guide* (rip.org.uk/publications/handbooks/teams/teamwork.pdf).

Austin, C. & Herbert, S.I. (1995) Clinical guidelines: should we be worried? *British Journal of Occupational Therapy* **58**(11), 481–484.

Backman, C. (2005) Outcomes and outcome measures: measuring what matters is in the eye of the beholder. *Canadian Journal of Occupational Therapy* **72**(5), 259–264.

Bailey, D.M. (1991) *Research for the Health Professional*. Philadelphia: FA Davis Co.

Bailey, D.M. (1997) *Research for the Health Professional*, 2nd edn. Philadelphia: FA Davis Co.

Baker, R., Dowling, Z., Wareing, L.A., Dawson, J. & Assey, J. (1997) Snoezelen: its long-term effects on older people with dementia. *British Journal of Occupational Therapy* **60**(5), 213–218.

Barbour, R.S. (2000) The role of qualitative research in broadening the 'evidence base' of clinical practice. *Journal of Evaluation in Clinical Practice* **6**, 155–163.

Barbour, R.S. (2001) Checklists for improving rigour in qualitative research: a case of the tail wagging the dog? *British Medical Journal* **322**, 1115–1117.

Barras, S. (2005) A systematic and critical review of the literature: the effectiveness of occupational therapy home assessment on a range of outcome measures. *Australian Occupational Therapy Journal* **52**, 326–336.

Bennett, S. & Bennett, J.W. (2000) The process of evidence-based practice in occupational therapy: informing clinical decisions. *Australian Occupational Therapy Journal* **47**, 171–180.

Bennett, K.J., Sackett, D.L., Haynes, R.B., Neufeld, V.R., Tugwell, P. & Roberts, R. (1987) A controlled trial of teaching critical appraisal of the clinical literature to medical students. *Journal of the American Medical Association* **257**(18), 2451–2454.

Bero, L.A., Grilli, R., Grimshaw, J., Harvey, E., Oxman, A.D. & Thomson, M.A. (1998) Closing the gap between research and practice: an overview of systematic reviews of interventions to promote the implementation of research findings. *British Medical Journal* **317**, 465–468.

Blair, S.E.E. & Robertson, L.J. (2005) Hard complexities – soft complexities: an exploration of philosophical positions related to evidence in occupational therapy. *British Journal of Occupational Therapy* **68**(6), 269–276.

Bowling, A. (2001) *Measuring Disease: A Review of Disease-specific Quality of Life Measurement Scales.* Buckingham: Open University Press.

Bowling, A. (2004) *Measuring Health: A Review of Quality of Life Measurement Scales*, 3rd edn. Buckingham: Open University Press.

British Journal of Therapy and Rehabilitation (1996) Supplement on evidence-based practice and mental health. *British Journal of Therapy and Rehabilitation* **3**(12), 659–670.

Broughton, R. & Rathbone, B. (2003) *What Makes a Good Clinical Guideline?* Hayward Medical Communications (http://www.evidence-based-medicine.co.uk/ebmfiles/WhatMakesClinGuide.pdf).

Brown, G.T. (1998) Research utilization: a purposeful activity for occupational therapists. Paper presentation. *12th International Congress of the World Federation of Occupational Therapists, Montreal.*

Brown, G.T. & Rodger, S. (1999) Research utilization models: frameworks for implementing evidence-based occupational therapy practice. *Occupational Therapy International* **6**(1), 1–23.

Brown, G.T., Brown, A. & Roever, C. (2005) Paediatric occupational therapy university programme curricula in the United Kingdom. *British Journal of Occupational Therapy* **68**(10), 457–466.

Bury, T. (1998) Getting research into practice: changing behaviour. In: Bury, T. & Mead, J. (eds) *Evidence-based Healthcare.* Oxford: Butterworth-Heinemann, pp. 66–84.

Buttery, Y. (1996) Implementing evidence through clinical audit. In: Bury, T. & Mead, J. (eds) *Evidence-based Healthcare.* Oxford: Butterworth-Heinemann, pp. 182–207.

Cameron, K.A.V., Ballantyne, S., Kulbitsky, A., Margolis-Gal, M., Daugherty, T. & Ludwig, F. (2005) Utilization of evidence-based practice by registered occupational therapists. *Occupational Therapy International* **12**(3), 123–136.

Canadian Association of Occupational Therapists (1991a) *Occupational Therapy Guidelines for Client-centred Practice.* Toronto: Canadian Association of Occupational Therapists.

Canadian Association of Occupational Therapists (1991b) *Enabling Occupation: an Occupational Therapy Perspective.* Ottawa: Canadian Association of Occupational Therapists.

Canadian Association of Occupational Therapists (1998) Special edition on evidence-based practice. *Canadian Journal of Occupational Therapy* **65**(3).

Canadian Association of Occupational Therapists, Association of Canadian Occupational Therapy University Programs, Association of Canadian Occupational Therapy Regulatory Organizations and the Presidents' Advisory Committee (1999) Joint position statement on evidence-based practice. *Canadian Journal of Occupational Therapy* **66**, 267–269.

Canadian Association of Occupational Therapists (2003) Special edition on evidence-based practice. *Canadian Journal of Occupational Therapy* **71**(4).

Canadian Task Force on the Periodic Health Examination (1979) The periodic health examination. *Canadian Medical Association Journal* **121**, 1193–1254.

Carlson, M., Fanchiang, S.P., Zemke, R. & Clark, F. (1996) A meta-analysis of the effectiveness of occupational therapy for older persons. *American Journal of Occupational Therapy* **50**(2), 89–98.

Chard, G. (2006) Adopting the Assessment of Motor and Process Skills into practice: therapists' voices. *British Journal of Occupational Therapy* **69**(2), 50–57.

Chartered Society of Physiotherapy (1996) *Literature Searching: Where to Go & What to Look For.* London: Chartered Society of Physiotherapy.

Chilvers, R., Harrison, G., Sipos, A. & Barley, M. (2002) Application of psychological models of change in evidence-based implementation. *British Journal of Psychiatry* **181**, 99–101.

Clegg, A. & Bannigan, K. (1997) Shifting the balance of opinion: RCTs in occupational therapy. *British Journal of Occupational Therapy* **60**, 510–512.

Clemence, M.L. (1998) Evidence-based physiotherapy: seeking the unattainable? *British Journal of Therapy and Rehabilitation* **5**(5), 257–260.

Cochrane, A. (1972) *Effectiveness and Efficiency.* London: Nuffield Provincial Hospitals Trust.

College of Occupational Therapists (1990) *Guidelines for Documentation.* London: College of Occupational Therapists.

College of Occupational Therapists (1997) Special edition on evidence-based practice. *British Journal of Occupational Therapy* **60**(11).

College of Occupational Therapists (2003) *Professional Standards for Occupational Therapy Practice.* London: College of Occupational Therapists.

College of Occupational Therapists (2004) *Practice Guidelines Development Manual.* London: College of Occupational Therapists.

College of Occupational Therapists (2005) *Code of Ethics and Professional Conduct.* London: College of Occupational Therapists.

Coolican, H. (1994) *Research Methods and Statistics in Psychology.* London: Hodder & Stoughton.

Cooper, E.J. (1995) Does the Rivermead Extended ADL Score indicate a patient's level of independence after discharge? BSc Dissertation, Oxford Brookes University, Oxford.

Craik, J. & Rappolt, S. (2003) Theory of research utilization enhancement: a model for occupational therapy. *Canadian Journal of Occupational Therapy* **70**(5), 266–275.

Creswell, J.W. (1998) *Qualitative Inquiry and Research Design: Choosing Among Five Traditions.* Thousand Oaks, CA: Sage.

Crombie, I.K. (1996) *The Pocket Guide to Critical Appraisal.* London: BMJ Publishing Group.

Curtin M. & Jaramazovic, E. (2001) Occupational therapists' views and perceptions of evidence-based practice. *British Journal of Occupational Therapy* **64**, 214–222.

Cusick, A. (1986) Research in occupational therapy: meta-analysis. *Australian Occupational Therapy Journal* **33**(4), 142–147.

Cusick, A. (2001) OZ OT EBP 21c: Australian occupational therapy, evidence-based practice and the 21st century. *Australian Occupational Therapy Journal* **48**(3), 102–117.

Dale, P. (ed.) (2000) *Guide to Libraries and Information Sources in Medicine and Health Care,* 3rd edn. London: The British Library.

Deane, K.H.O., Ellis-Hill, C., Clarke, C.E., Playford, D. & Ben-Shlomo, Y. (2001) Occupational therapy for Parkinson's disease (Cochrane review). *Cochrane Database of Systematic Reviews* CD002813. Chichester: Wiley Interscience.

Deane, K.H.O., Ellis-Hill, C., Dekker, K., Davies, P. & Clarke, C.E. (2003a) A survey of current occupational therapy practice for Parkinson's disease in the United Kingdom. *British Journal of Occupational Therapy* **66**(5), 193–200.

Deane, K.H.O., Ellis-Hill, C., Dekker, K., Davies, P. & Clarke, C.E. (2003b) A Delphi survey of best practice occupational therapy for Parkinson's disease in the United Kingdom. *British Journal of Occupational Therapy* **66**(6), 247–254.

Denzin, N.K. & Lincoln, Y.S. (1994) Introduction: entering the field of qualitative research. In: Denzin, N.K. & Lincoln, Y.S. (eds) *Handbook of Qualitative Research*. Thousand Oaks, CA: Sage, pp. 1–17.

Department of Health (1991) *Audit for Nursing and Therapy Professions in HCHS: Allocation of Funds 1991/92*. PL/CNO (91/3). London: Department of Health.

Department of Health (1997) *The New NHS: Modern-Dependable*. London: HMSO.

Department of Health (1998a) *A First Class Service: Quality in the New NHS*. London: Department of Health.

Department of Health (1998b). *Modernising Social Services*. London: Department of Health.

DePoy, E. & Gitlin, L.N. (2005) *Introduction to Research*, 3rd edn. St Louis: Mosby.

Droogan, J. & Bannigan, K. (1997) A review of psychosocial family interventions for schizophrenia. *Nursing Times* **93**(26), 46–47.

Dubouloz, C.J., Egan, M., Vallerand, J. & von Zweck, C. (1999) Occupational therapists' perceptions of evidence-based practice. *American Journal of Occupational Therapy* **53**(5), 445–453.

Dunning, M., Abi-Aad, G., Gilbert, D., Gillam, S. & Livett, H. (1998) *Turning Evidence into Everyday Practice*. London: King's Fund.

Eriksson, G., Tham, K. & Borg, J. (2006) Occupational gaps in everyday life 1–4 years after acquired brain injury. *Journal of Rehabilitation Medicine* **38**, 159–165.

Eysenbach, G. & Köhler, C. (2002) How do consumers search for and appraise health information on the world wide web? Qualitative study using focus groups, usability tests, and in-depth interviews. *British Medical Journal* **324**, 573–577.

Eysenck, H.J. (1978) An exercise in mega-silliness. *American Psychologist* **33**, 517.

Fearing, V.G., Law, M. & Clark, J. (1997) An occupational performance process model: fostering client and therapists alliances. *Canadian Journal of Occupational Therapy* **64**(1), 7–15.

Finlay, L. (1997) Good patients and bad patients: how occupational therapists view their patients/clients. *British Journal of Occupational Therapy* **60**(10), 440–446.

Finlay, L. (1998) Reflexivity: an essential component of all research? *British Journal of Occupational Therapy* **61**(10), 453–456.

Gabbay, J. & le May, A. (2004) Evidence based guidelines or collectively constructed 'mindlines'? Ethnographic study of knowledge management in primary care. *British Medical Journal* **329**, 1013–1017.

Gitlin, L., Corcoran, M., Winter, L., Boyce, A. & Hauck, W.W. (2001) A randomised, controlled trial of a home environmental intervention: effect on efficacy and upset in caregivers and on daily function of persons with dementia. *The Gerontologist* **41**(1), 4–14.

Goodacre, L. (2006) Women's perceptions on managing chronic arthritis. *British Journal of Occupational Therapy* **69**(1), 7–14.

Gräsel, E., Biehler, J., Schmidt, R. & Schupp, W. (2005) Intensification of the transition between inpatient neurological rehabilitation and home care of stroke patients. Controlled clinical trial with follow-up assessment six months after discharge. *Clinical Rehabilitation* **19**, 725–736.

Gray, J.A.M. (2001) *Evidence-based Healthcare*, 2nd edn. Edinburgh: Churchill Livingstone.

Green, S. & Higgins, J. (eds) (2005) *Cochrane Handbook for Systematic Reviews of Interventions 4.2.5* [updated May 2005] (http://www.cochrane.uk/cochrane/handbook/handbook.htm).

Greenhalgh, T. (2006) *How to Read a Paper,* 3rd edn. Oxford: Blackwell Publishing.

Greenhalgh, T., Robert, G., Macfarlane, F., Bate, P., Kyriakidou, O. & Peacock, R. (2005) Storylines of research in diffusion of innovation: a meta-narrative approach to systematic reviews. *Social Science and Medicine* **61**, 417–430.

Greyson, L. (1997) *Evidence-based Medicine.* London: The British Library.

Grimley Evans, J. (1995) Evidence-based and evidence-biased medicine. *Age and Ageing* **24**, 461–463.

Grimshaw, J. & Russell, I.T. (1993) Effect of clinical guidelines on medical practice. A systematic review of rigorous evaluations. *Lancet* **342**, 1317–1322.

Grol, R., Dalhuijsen, J., Thomas, S., Veld, C., Rutten, G. & Mokkink, H. (1998) Attributes of clinical guidelines that influence use of guidelines in general practice: observational study. *British Medical Journal* **317**, 858–861.

Haddon-Silver, A. (1993) Homophobia amongst OT students: issues, incidence and implications. BSc Dissertation. Oxford Brookes University, Oxford.

Hammersley, M. (1990) *Reading Ethnographic Research*. New York: Longman.

Hammond, A., Young, A. & Kidao, R. (2004) A randomised controlled trial of occupational therapy for people with early rheumatoid arthritis. *Annals of the Rheumatic Diseases* **63**(1), 23–30.

Hansen, R., Tresse, S. & Gunnarsson, J. (2004) Fewer accidents and better maintenance with active wheelchair check-ups: a randomized controlled clinical trial. *Clinical Rehabilitation* **18**, 631–639.

Hasselkus, B.R. (1992) The meaning of activity: day care for persons with Alzheimer disease. *American Journal of Occupational Therapy* **46**, 199–206.

Health Professions Council (2003) *Standards of Proficiency, Occupational Therapists.* London: Health Professions Council.

Herbert, R., Jamtvedt, G., Mead, J. & Hagen, K.B. (2005) *Practical Evidence-based Physiotherapy*. Edinburgh: Churchill Livingstone.

Hocking, C. & Ness, N.E. (2002) *Revised Minimum Standards for the Education of Occupational Therapists.* Perth: World Federation of Occupational Therapists.

Hopewell, S., Clarke, M., Lefebvre, C. & Scherer, R. (2004) Handsearching versus electronic searching to identify reports of randomized trials (Cochrane Methodology review). *The Cochrane Library*, issue 1, 2005. Chichester: John Wiley & Sons.

Hyde, P. (2004) Fool's gold: examining the use of gold standards in the production of research evidence. *British Journal of Occupational Therapy* **67**(2), 89–94.

Jadad, A.R., Moore, R.A., Caroll, D. *et al.* (1996) Assessing the quality of reports of randomised clinical trials: is blinding necessary? *Controlled Clinical Trials* **17**, 1–12.

Jerosch-Herold, C. (2005) An evidence-based approach to choosing outcome measures: a checklist for the critical appraisal of validity, reliability and responsiveness studies. *British Journal of Occupational Therapy* **68**(8), 347–353.

Kearney, M.H. (2001) Levels and application of qualitative research evidence. *Research in Nursing and Health* **24**, 145–153.

Keep, J. (1998) Change management. In: Bury, T. & Mead, J. (eds) *Evidence-based Healthcare*. Oxford: Butterworth-Heinemann, pp. 45–65.

Kielhofner, G. (1982) Qualitative research: part two, methodological approaches and relevance to occupational therapy. *Occupational Therapy Journal of Research* **2**, 150–170.

Kiley, R. (2003) *Medical Information on the Internet*. Edinburgh: Churchill Livingstone.

Kloczko, E. & Ikiugu, M.N. (2006) The role of occupational therapy in the treatment of adolescents with eating disorders as perceived by mental health therapists. *Occupational Therapy in Mental Health* **22**(1), 63–83.

Knott, J. & Wildavsky, A. (1980) If dissemination is the solution, what is the problem? *Knowledge, Creation, Diffusion, Utilization* **1**(4), 537–578.

Kogan, M., Redfern, S., Kober, A. *et al.* (1995) *Making Use of Clinical Audit: A Guide to Practice in the Health Professions*. Buckingham: Open University Press.

Krefting, L. (1989a) Disability ethnography: a methodological approach for occupational therapy. *Canadian Journal of Occupational Therapy* **56**(2), 61–66.

Krefting, L.M. (1989b) Reintegration into the community after head injury: the results of an ethnographic study. *Occupational Therapy Journal of Research* **9**, 67–83.

Krefting, L. (1991) Rigor in qualitative research: the assessment of trustworthiness. *American Journal of Occupational Therapy* **45**(3), 214–222.

Kylma, J. (2005) Hope, despair and hopelessness in significant others of adult persons living with HIV. *Journal of Theory Construction and Testing* **9**(2), 49–54.

Langhorne, P. & Dennis, M. (1998) *Stroke Units: an Evidence Based Approach*. London: BMJ Publishing Group.

Langhorne, P., Wagenaar, R. & Partridge, C. (1996) Physiotherapy after stroke: more is better? *Physiotherapy Research International* **1**(2), 75–88.

Law, M. (ed.) (1998) *Client-centered Occupational Therapy*. Thorofare, NJ: Slack.

Law, M. (ed.) (2002) *Evidence-based Rehabilitation: a Guide to Practice*. Thorofare, NJ: Slack.

Law, M., Stewart, D., Letts, L., Pollock, N., Bosch, J. & Westmorland, M. (1998) *Critical Review Form – Qualitative and Quantitative Studies*. Hamilton: McMaster University.

Law, M., Baum, C. & Dunn, W. (2001) *Measuring Occupational Performance*. Thorofare, NJ: Slack Incorporated.

Liddle, J., March, L., Carfrae, B. *et al.* (1996) Can occupational therapy intervention play a part in maintaining independence and quality of life in older people? A randomised controlled trial. *Australian and New Zealand Journal of Public Health* **20**(6), 574–578.

Liepold, A. & Mathiowetz, V. (2005) Reliability and validity of the Self-Efficacy for Performing Energy Conservation Strategies Assessment for persons with multiple sclerosis. *Occupational Therapy International* **12**(3), 234–249.

Lin, K., Wu, C., Tickle-Degnen, L. & Coster, W. (1997) Enhancing occupational performance through occupationally embedded exercise: a meta-analytic review. *Occupational Therapy Journal of Research* **17**(1), 25–47.

Lincoln, Y.S. & Guba, E.A. (1985) *Naturalistic Inquiry.* Beverly Hills: Sage.

Linzer, M. (1987) The journal club and medical education: over one hundred years of unrecorded history. *Postgraduate Medical Journal* **63**, 475–378.

Linzer, M., Brown, T., Frazier, L. *et al.* (1988) Impact of a medical journal on house-staff reading habits, knowledge and critical appraisal skills. *Journal of the American Medical Association* **260**, 2537–2541.

Littlewood, S.A. (1997) Do OT students consider sexual orientation when implementing treatment? BSc Dissertation. Oxford Brookes University, Oxford.

Logan, P.A., Ahern, J., Gladman, J.R. & Lincoln, N.B. (1997) A randomized controlled trial of enhanced Social Services occupational therapy for stroke patients. *Clinical Rehabilitation* **11**(2), 107–113.

MacAuley, D. & McGram, E. (1999) Critical appraisal using the READER method: a workshop based controlled trial. *Family Practice* **16**, 90–93.

McClarey, M. & Thompson, J. (2000) Clinical guidelines and the law. *Health Care Risk Report* **6**(4), 19–20.

McCluskey, A. & Cusick, A. (2002) Strategies for introducing evidence-based practice and changing clinician behaviour: a manager's toolbox. *Australian Occupational Therapy Journal* **49**, 63–70.

McCluskey, A., Lovarini, M., Bennett, S., McKenna, K., Tooth, L. & Hoffmann, T. (2006) How and why do occupational therapists use the OTseeker evidence database? *Australian Occupational Therapy Journal* **53**, 188–195.

McCuaig, M. & Frank, G. (1991) The able self: adaptive patterns and choices in independent living for a person with cerebral palsy. *American Journal of Occupational Therapy* **45**(3), 224–234.

McKenna, K., Bennett, S., Dierslhuis, Z., Hoffman, T., Tooth, L. & McCluskey, A. (2005) Australian occupational therapists' use of an online evidence-based practice database (OTSeeker). *Health Information & Libraries Journal* **22**, 205–214.

McKinnell, I. & Elliott, J. (1997) *The Cochrane Library: Self-Training Guide and Notes.* Oxford: NHS Executive Anglia & Oxford (http://www.york.ac.uk/inst/crd/cochlib.htm).

Maher, C.G., Sherrington, C., Herbert, R.D., Moseley, A.M. & Elkins, M. (2003) Reliability of the PEDro Scale for rating quality of randomized controlled trials. *Physical Therapy* **83**(8), 713–721.

Malby, R. (1995) *Clinical Audit for Nurses and Therapists.* London: Scutari.

Mann, T. (1996) *Clinical Guidelines: Using Clinical Guidelines to Improve Patient Care within the NHS.* London: Department of Health.

Mathiowetz, V.G., Finlayson, M.L., Matuska, K.M., Hua, Y.C. & Ping Luo, P. (2005) Randomised controlled trial of an energy conservation course for persons with multiple sclerosis. *Multiple Sclerosis* **11**, 592–601.

Mattingly, C. & Fleming, M.H. (1994) *Clinical Reasoning: Forms of Inquiry in a Therapeutic Practice.* Philadelphia: F.A. Davis.

Mays, N. & Pope, C. (2000) Assessing quality in qualitative research. *British Medical Journal* **320**, 50–52.

Middleton, S., Barnett, J. & Reeves, D. (2003) *What is an Integrated Care Pathway?* Hayward Medical Communications (http://www.evidence-based-medicine.co.uk/ebmfiles/WhatisanICP.pdf).

Missiuna, C., Moll, S., Law, M., King, S. & King, G. (2006) Mysteries and mazes; parents' experiences of children with developmental coordination disorder. *Canadian Journal of Occupational Therapy* **73**(1), 7–17.

Moher, D., Jadad, A., Nichol, G. *et al.* (1995) Assessing the quality of randomized controlled trials: an annotated bibliography of scales and checklists. *Controlled Clinical Trials* **16**, 62–73.

Montori, V.M., Wilczynski, N.L., Morgan, D., Haynes, R.B. & the Hedges Team (2005) Optimal search strategies for retrieving systematic reviews from Medline: analytical survey. *British Medical Journal* **330**, 68–73.

Moreton, S. (1998) Local clinical guidelines – can they make us better? Paper presentation. *World Federation of Occupational Therapists 12th World Congress,* Montreal.

Morse, J.M., Hutchinson, S.A. & Penrod, J. (1998) From theory to practice: the development of assessment guides from qualitatively derived theory. *Qualitative Health Research* **8**, 329–340.

Mulrow, C.D. (1994) Rationale for systematic reviews. *British Medical Journal* **309**, 597–599.

Murphy, M.K., Black, N.A., Lamping, D.L. *et al.* (1998) Consensus development methods, and their use in clinical guideline development. *Health Technology Assessment* **2**, i–88.

National Association of Rheumatology Occupational Therapists (2003) *Occupational Therapy Clinical Guidelines for Rheumatology*. London: College of Occupational Therapists.

National Collaborating Centre for Chronic Conditions (2004) *Multiple Sclerosis: National Clinical Guideline for Diagnosis and Management in Primary and Secondary Care*. London: Royal College of Physicians.

Needham, G. & Oliver, S. (1998) Involving service users. In: Bury, T. & Mead, J. (eds) *Evidence-based Healthcare*. Oxford: Butterworth-Heinemann, pp. 85–104.

Newell, R. (1997) Towards clinical effectiveness in nursing. *Clinical Effectiveness in Nursing* **1**(1), 1–2.

New Zealand Guidelines Group (2001) *Handbook for the Preparation of Explicit Evidence-based Clinical Practice Guidelines*. Wellington: New Zealand Guidelines Group.

NHS CRD (2001) *Undertaking Systematic Reviews of Research on Effectiveness: CRD's Guidance to Those Carrying out or Commissioning Reviews*. CRD Report 4, 2nd edn. York: Centre for Reviews and Dissemination, University of York.

NHS Executive (1996) *Promoting Clinical Effectiveness: A Framework for Action*. Leeds: NHS Executive.

NHS Executive (1998) *Information for Health: An Information Strategy for the Modern NHS 1998–2005. A National Strategy for Local Implementation*. Leeds/London: Department of Health.

NHS Management Executive (1994) *Clinical Audit: 1994/95 and Beyond*. EL(94)20. London: Department of Health.

Oppenheim, A.N. (1992) *Questionnaire Design, Interviewing and Attitude Measurement*. Thousand Oaks, CA: Sage.

Ottenbacher, K. (1983) Quantitative reviewing: the literature review as scientific inquiry. *American Journal of Occupational Therapy* **37**(5), 313–319.

Ottenbacher, K.J. & Maas, F. (1999) How to detect effects: statistical power and evidence-based practice in occupational therapy research. *American Journal of Occupational Therapy* **53**(2), 181–188.

Pain, K., Magill-Evans, J., Darrah, J., Hagler, P. & Warren, S. (2004) Effects of profession and facility type on research utlization by rehabilitation professionals. *Journal of Allied Health* **33**(1), 3–9.

Pawson, R., Boaz, A., Grayson, L., Long, A. & Barnes, C. (2003) *Knowledge Reviews 3: Types and Quality of Knowledge in Social Care*. London: SCIE & The Policy Press.

Pereira-Maxwell, F. (1998) *A–Z of Medical Statistics*. London: Arnold.

Peterson, G., Aslani, P. & Williams, K.A. (2003) How do consumers search for and appraise information on medicines on the internet? A qualitative study using focus groups. *Journal of Medical Internet Research* **5**(4), e33.

Petticrew, M. (2001) Systematic reviews from astronomy to zoology: myths and misconceptions. *British Medical Journal* **322**, 98–101.

Petticrew, M. & Roberts, H. (2006) *Systematic Reviews in the Social Sciences*. Oxford: Blackwell Publishing.

Phillips, B., Ball, C. & Sackett, D. *et al.* (2001) *Oxford Centre for Evidence-based Medicine Levels of Evidence (May 2001)*, http://www.cebm.net/levels_of_evidence.asp.

Piercy, M. (1998) An audit of the reliability of the Frenchay Activities Index. BSc Dissertation. Oxford Brookes University, Oxford.

Piergrossi, J. (2004) A question of priorities: notes from the International Conference on Evidence-based Occupational Therapy, July 11–14, 2005, Washington D.C., USA. *World Federation of Occupational Therapists Bulletin* **50**, 48–50.

Pollock, A.S., Legg, L., Langhorne, P. & Sellars, C. (2000) Barriers to achieving evidence-based stroke rehabilitation. *Clinical Rehabilitation* **14**, 611–617.

Popay, J. & Williams, G. (1998) Qualitative research and evidence-based healthcare. *Journal of the Royal Society of Medicine* **91** (Suppl. 35), 32–37.

Popay, J., Rogers, A. & Williams, G. (1998) Rationale and standards for the systematic review of qualitative literature in health services research. *Journal of Qualitative Health Research* **8**, 341–351.

Pope, C. & Mays, N. (2006) *Qualitative Research in Health Care*, 3rd edn. Oxford: Blackwell Publishing.

Powell, J.A., Darvell, M. & Gray, J.A.M. (2003) The doctor, the patient and the world-wide web: how the internet is changing healthcare. *Journal of the Royal Society of Medicine* **96**, 74–76.

Pringle, E. (1999) EBP: is it for me? *Therapy Weekly* **25**(46), 12.

Prochaska, J.O. & DiClemente, C.C. (1982) Transtheoretical therapy: towards a more integrative model of change. *Psychotherapy: Theory, Research and Practice* **20**, 161–173.

Prochaska, J.O., DiClemente, C.C. & Norcross, J.C. (1992) In search of how people change. *American Psychologist* **47**(9), 1102–1114.

Przybylski, B.R., Dumont, E.D., Watkins, M.E., Warren, S.A., Beaulne, A.P. & Lier, D.A. (1996) Outcomes of enhanced physical and occupational therapy service in a nursing home setting. *Archives of Physical Medicine and Rehabilitation* **77**(6), 554–561.

Rappolt, S. (2003) The role of professional expertise in evidence-based occupational therapy. *American Journal of Occupational Therapy* **57**(5), 589–593.

Reynard, K.W. & Reynard, J.M.E. (eds) (1996) *ASLIB Directory of Information Services in the United Kingdom.* London: ASLIB.

Richardson, W.S., Wilson, M.C., Nishikawa, J. *et al.* (1995) The well-built clinical question: a key to evidence-based decisions (editorial). *ACP Journal Club* **123**, A12–A13.

Risk, A. (2002) Commentary: on the way to quality. *British Medical Journal* **324**, 601.

Risk, A, & Petersen, C. (2002) Health information on the internet: quality issues and international initiatives. *JAMA* **287**(20), 213–217.

Rogers, E. (1983) *Diffusion of Innovation.* New York: Free Press.

Rosenberg, W. & Donald, A. (1995) Evidence based medicine: an approach to clinical problem-solving. *British Medical Journal* **310**, 1122–1126.

Rycroft-Malone, J., Harvey, G., Seers, K., Kitson, A., McCormack, B. & Titchen, A. (2004) An exploration of the factors that influence the implementation of evidence into practice. *Journal of Clinical Nursing* **13**, 913–924.

Sackett, D.L. (19 March 1998). *Shamanism (Was: Pre-test probability).* Evidence-based-health [online]. Available from: http://www.jiscmail.ac.uk/ [8 June 2000]

Sackett, D.L. & Wennberg, J.E. (1997) Choosing the best research design for each question. *British Medical Journal* **315**, 1636.

Sackett, D.L., Rosenberg, W.M.C., Gray, J.A.M., Haynes, R.B. & Richardson, W.S. (1996) Evidence-based medicine: what it is and what it isn't. *British Medical Journal* **312**, 71–72.

Sackett, D.L., Richardson, W.S., Rosenberg, W. & Hayes, R.B. (1997) *Evidence-based Medicine: How to Practice and Teach EBM.* New York: Churchill Livingstone.

Sackett, D.L., Strauss, S.E., Richardson, W.S., Rosenberg, W.M.C. & Haynes, R.B. (2000) *Evidence-based Medicine: How to Practice and Teach EBM,* 2nd edn. Edinburgh: Churchill Livingstone.

Sale, D. (1996) *Quality Assurance for Nurses and Other Members of the Health Care Team.* London: Macmillan.

Savin-Baden, M. & Fisher, A. (2002) Negotiating 'honesties' in the research process. *British Journal of Occupational Therapy* **65**(4), 191–193.

Scottish Intercollegiate Guidelines Network (2002) *A Guideline Developers' Handbook.* Edinburgh: Scottish Intercollegiate Guidelines Network.

Sellar, B. & Boshoff, K. (2006) Subjective leisure experiences of older Australians. *Australian Occupational Therapy Journal* **53**, 211–219.

Shaw, A., Joseph, S. & Linley, P.A. (2005) Religion, spirituality, and posttraumatic growth: a systematic review. *Mental Health, Religion & Culture* **8**(1), 1–11.

Shin, J.H., Haynes, R.B. & Johnston, M.E. (1993) Effect of problem-based, self-directed undergraduate education on life-long learning. *Canadian Medical Association Journal* **148**(6), 969–976.

Shopland, A.J., Hardial, P.M., Unwin, A.M., Vickers, S.M., Westmore, V.R. & Williams, A.J. (1975) *Refer to Occupational Therapy.* Edinburgh: Churchill Livinstone.

Spector, A. & Orrell, M. (1998a) Reminiscence therapy for dementia: a review of the evidence of effectiveness (Cochrane review). *The Cochrane Library*, issue 3, 1998. Oxford: Update Software.

Spector, A. & Orrell, M. (1998b) Reality orientation for dementia: a review of the evidence of effectiveness (Cochrane review). *The Cochrane Library*, issue 3, 1998. Oxford: Update Software.

Spencer, J., Young, M., Rintala, D. & Bates, S. (1995) Socialization to the culture of a rehabilitation hospital: an ethnographic study. *American Journal of Occupational Therapy* **49**(1), 53–62.

Spencer, L., Ritchie, J., Lewis, J. & Dillon, L. (2003) *Quality in Qualitative Evaluation: a Framework for Assessing Research Evidence.* London: Government Chief Social Researcher's Office.

Steultjens, E.M.J., Dekker, J., Bouter, L.M., van Schaardenburg, D., van Kuyk, M.A.H. & van den Ende, C.H.M. (2004) Occupational therapy for rheumatoid arthritis. *Cochrane Database of Systematic Reviews*, issue 1, CD003114, doi: 10.1002/14651858.CD003114.pub2.

Steultjens, E.M.J., Dekker, J., Bouter, L.M., Leemrijse, C.J. & van den Ende, C.H. (2005) Evidence of the efficacy of occupational therapy in different conditions: an overview of systematic reviews. *Clinical Rehabilitation* **19**(3), 247–254.

Stewart, S., Harvey, I., Poland, F., Lloyd-Smith, W., Mugford, M. & Flood, C. (2005) Are occupational therapists more effective than social workers when assessing frail older people? Results of CAMELOT, a randomised controlled trial. *Age and Ageing* **34**(1), 41–46.

Strauss, S.E., Richardson, W.S., Glasziou, P. & Haynes, R.B. (2005) *Evidence-based Medicine: How to Practice and Teach EBM*, 3rd edn. Edinburgh: Churchill Livingstone.

Sumsion, T. (1997) Client-centred implications of evidence-based practice. *Physiotherapy* **83**(7), 373–374.

Swinglehurst, D. (2005) Evidence-based guidelines: the theory and the practice. *Evidence Based Medicine and Public Health* **9**, 308–314.

Taylor, M.C. (1997) What is evidence-based practice? *British Journal of Occupational Therapy* **60**(11), 470–474.

Taylor, M.C. (1999) The devil makes work for idle hands – reviewing the evidence for the value of 'activity' as an intervention for depression. Conference Presentation. *Second Evidence-based Mental Health Conference*, Norwich.

Taylor, M.C. (2000) *Evidence-based Practice for Occupational Therapists.* Oxford: Blackwell Science.

Taylor, M.C. (2003) Evidence-based practice: informing practice and critically evaluating related research. In: Brown, G., Esdaile, S.A. & Ryan, S.E. (eds) *Becoming an Advanced Healthcare Practitioner.* Edinburgh: Butterworth-Heinemann, pp. 90–117.

Taylor, L.P. & McGruder, J.E. (1996) The meanings of sea kayaking for persons with spinal cord injuries. *American Journal of Occupational Therapy* **50**(1), 39–46.

Thomas, L., Cullum, N., McColl, E., Rousseau, N., Soutter, J. & Steen N. (1999) Clinical guidelines in nursing, midwifery and other professions allied to medicine (Cochrane review). *The Cochrane Library*, issue 1, 1999. Oxford: Update Software.

Thomas, J., Harden, A., Oakley, A. *et al.* (2004) Integrating qualitative research with trials in systematic reviews. *British Medical Journal* **328**, 1010–1012.

Thurston, N.E. & King, K.M. (2004) Implementing evidence-based practice: walking the talk. *Applied Nursing Research* **17**(4), 239–247.

Tickle-Degnen, L. (1998) Communicating with clients about treatment outcomes: the use of meta-analytic evidence in collaborative treatment planning. *American Journal of Occupational Therapy* **52**(7), 526–530.

Townsend, E. (1996) Institutional ethnography: a method of showing how the context shapes practice. *Occupational Therapy Journal of Research* **16**(3), 179–199.

Tse, T. (2005) The environment and falls prevention: do environmental modifications make a difference? *Australian Occupational Therapy Journal* **52**, 271–281.

Tse, S., Blackwood, K. & Marrolee, P. (2000) From rhetoric to reality: use of randomised controlled trials in evidence-based occupational therapy. *Australian Occupational Therapy Journal* **47**(4), 181–185.

Turner, P.A. & Whitefield, T.W. (1996) A multivariate analysis of physiotherapy clinicians' journal readership. *Physiotherapy Theory and Practice* **12**(4), 221–223.

Turner, P. & Whitefield, T.W. (1997) Journal readership amongst Australian physiotherapists: a cross-national replication. *Australian Journal of Physiotherapy* **43**(3), 197–202.

UK Health Centre (2002) *Guidance on Assessing Health and Medical Information on the Internet.* UK Health Centre (www.healthcentre.org.uk/hc/index.html).

Upton, D. (1999a) Clinical effectiveness and EBP 2: attitudes of health-care professionals. *British Journal of Therapy and Rehabilitation* **6**(1), 26–30.

Upton, D. (1999b) Clinical effectiveness and EBP 3: application by health-care professionals. *British Journal of Therapy and Rehabilitation* **6**(2), 86–90.

Van Tulder, M.W., Assendelft, W.J.J., Koes, B.W. & Bouter, L.M. (1997) Method guidelines for systematic reviews in the Cochrane Collaboration back review group for spinal disorders. *Spine* **22**, 2323–2330.

de Vet, H.C.W., de Bie, R.A., van der Heijden, G.J.M.G, Verhagen, A.P., Sijpkes, P. & Knipschild, P.G. (1997) Systematic reviews on the basis of methodological criteria. *Physiotherapy* **83**(6), 284–298.

Wagstaff, S. (2005) Supports and barriers for exercise participation for well elders: implications for occupational therapy. *Physical and Occupational Therapy in Geriatrics* **24**(2), 19–33.

Walshe, K. (1998) Quality moves to the top of the agenda. *Health Service Management Centre Newsletter* **4**, 2.

Ward, C.D., Turpin, G., Dewey, M.E. *et al.* (2004) Education for people with progressive neurological conditions can have negative effects: evidence from a randomized controlled trial. *Clinical Rehabilitation* **18**, 717–725.

Welch, A. & Dawson, P. (2006) Closing the gap: collaborative learning as a strategy to embed evidence within occupational therapy practice. *Journal of Evaluation in Clinical Practice* **12**(2), 227–238.

Whitcher, K. & Tse, S. (2004) Counselling skills in occupational therapy: a grounded theory approach to explain their use within mental health in New Zealand. *British Journal of Occupational Therapy* **67**(8), 361–368.

Wiles, R. & Barnard, S. (1998) Physiotherapy and evidence-based practice. Paper presentation. *BSA Medical Sociology Group 30th Annual Conference: York.*

Wilson, P. (2002) How to find the good and avoid the bad or ugly: a short guide to tools for rating quality of health information on the internet. *British Medical Journal* **324**, 598–600.

Wilson-Barnett, J. (1998) Evidence for nursing practice – an overview. *NT Research* **3**(1), 12–14.

World Federation of Occupational Therapists (2004) *Code of Ethics for Occupational Therapists*. World Federation of Occupational Therapists (www.wfot.org).

Woodside, H., Schell, L. & Allison-Hedges, J. (2006) Listening to recovery: the vocational success of people living with mental illness. *Canadian Journal of Occupational Therapy* **73**(1), 36–43.

Yerxa, E.J. (1991) Seeking a relevant, ethical, and realistic way of knowing for occupational therapy. *American Journal of Occupational Therapy* **45**(3), 199–204.

Yuker, H.E., Block, J.R. & Campbell, W. (1960) *A Scale to Measure Attitudes Towards Disabled Persons*. New York: HRC.

Zisselman, M.H., Rovner, B.W., Shmuely, Y. & Ferrie, P. (1996) A pet therapy intervention with geriatric inpatients. *American Journal of Occupational Therapy* **50**(1), 47–51.

Index

AMED (Allied and Complementary
     Medicine Database), 22, 27–8, 30–4,
     36, 38, 86–7, 101, 168–9, 185
appraisal checklists,
   guidelines, 159–62
   internet-based evidence, 122–5
   outcome measures, 118–20
   qualitative research, 95–103
   RCTs, 53–65
   surveys, 109–14
   systematic reviews, 77–84
ASSIA (Applied Social Science Index of
     Abstracts), 22, 29–30, 36, 38, 168,
     169–70, 185
audit, 4, 93, 99
   comparison with evidence-based
     practice, 4–5
   comparison with research and evidence-
     based practice, 4–5
   definitions, 4
   evidence-based, 131–2, 142, 155

Bandolier, 182, 185
barriers, 134–7
bias, 55, 72–3
blinding, 47, 55, 57, 61, 63, 185
blobbogram, 75–6
books, 20, 181–3
Boolean operators, 24–5, 33, 87, 185

Campbell Collaboration, 86
CAPs (critically appraised papers), 139, 185
CASP (Critical Appraisal Skills
     Programme), 54, 77, 96, 136, 176, 186
CATs (critically appraised topics), 155, 178,
     186

Centre for Evidence-based Medicine, 176
change management, 140–2
   Transtheoretical Model of Change, 140,
     141, 143
CINAHL (Cumulative Index of Nursing
     and Allied Health Literature), 22,
     26, 35–6, 38, 43, 66–8, 79, 86–7, 106,
     168, 170, 186
citation tracking, 148, 150
client-centred practice, 133, 137
clinical effectiveness, 131–2, 134, 186
clinical guidelines, 131, 156–67, 186
clinical significance, 52–3, 66, 186
Cochrane Collaboration, 86, 186
Cochrane Library, 22, 24, 29–30, 36, 38,
     67–8, 79, 149, 171, 173, 186
   Cochrane Central Register of Controlled
     Trials, 29–30, 43, 79, 172, 186
   Cochrane Database of Systematic
     Reviews, 29–30, 67–8, 79, 171–2, 186
confidence interval (CI), 52–3, 187
confirmability, 93, 95, 101, 187
CONSORT statement, 54
continuing professional development
     (CPD), 135
control groups, 45–6, 187
controlled clinical trials (CCT), 15, 23, 38,
     46–7, 147, 187
credibility, 93–4, 99, 101, 187
critical appraisal, 53, 54, 129, 152, 187
   guidelines, 159–62
   outcome measures, 118–20
   qualitative research, 87, 95–103
   RCTs, 53–65
   surveys, 109–14
   systematic reviews, 77–84

websites, 122–5
critically appraised papers *see* CAPs
critically appraised topics *see* CATs

DARE (Database of Abstracts of Reviews
    of Effectiveness), 22, 24, 67, 79,
    172–3, 186–7
databases,
    AMED, 22, 27–8, 30–34, 36, 38, 86–7, 101,
        168–9, 185
    ASSIA, 22, 29–30, 36, 38, 168–70, 185
    CINAHL, 22, 26, 35–6, 38, 43, 66–8, 79,
        86–7, 106, 168, 170, 186
    Cochrane Library, 22, 24, 29–30, 36, 38,
        67–8, 79, 149, 171, 173, 186
    DARE, 22, 24, 79, 172–3, 186–7
    EMBASE, 22, 173
    ERIC, 22
    MEDLINE, 22, 37, 106, 168, 173, 178,
        188
    OTBIBSys, 22, 174, 189
    OTDBase, 22, 30–31, 37–8, 174–5, 189
    OTSeeker, 22, 24, 26, 37–8, 67, 106, 108,
        121, 149, 175, 189
    PEDro, 22, 121, 175, 189
    PubMed, 22, 27–8, 37–8, 178, 188–90
databases,
    information storage, 40–41
        Access, 41
        Endnote, 41
data extraction, 152–3, 187
dependability, 93, 95, 101, 187
descriptive statistics, 48–9
discussion lists, 179–80
    Critical Appraisal Skills, 180
    Evidence-based Health, 180
    Occup-ther, 180
    Occupational-therapy, 180

effectiveness, 106, 182, 187
EMBASE, 22, 173
ERIC, 22
ethnography, 87, 89–90, 188
evidence-based culture, 140–43
evidence-based medicine, 1–4
    definitions, 2, 4
    origins, 1
evidence-based occupational therapy,
    definition, 3–4

development, 2–4, 127
    process, 133
    stages of, 133
    web portal, 121–2, 177
evidence-based practice,
    comparison with audit and research,
        4–5
    comparison with research utilisation,
        138
    developing evidence-based questions,
        10–11, 147
    examples of evidence-based questions,
        12–14, 148
    stages of, 8

generalisability, 188
Google, 33, 35, 38, 106,
    Google Scholar, 177
grey literature, 6, 135, 148
grounded theory, 87, 91
guidelines, 131–2, 142, 156–67

hand searching, 69–70, 148–50
Hawthorne effect, 63
heterogeneity, 73, 81, 188
hierarchy of evidence, 16–17
homogeneity, 73, 188

inclusion criteria,
    in research, 47
    in systematic reviews, 70–2, 78–9, 151
inferential statistics, 49–52

journal clubs, 129–31, 142
journals, 7, 170, 173, 182
    evidence-based, 182
    hand searching, 69, 70, 148–50

levels of evidence, 15
librarians, 23, 39
literature searching, 23–39
    examples of, 25–35

MEDLINE, 22, 37, 106, 168, 173, 178, 188
mentoring, 128–9
MeSH (Medical Subject Heading) terms,
    24, 28, 30, 68, 189
meta analysis, 66, 74–7, 83, 153, 188–9

National Research Register (NRR), 174
NHS Centre for Reviews and
    Dissemination (NHS CRD), 152, 178
numbers needed to treat (NNT), 53, 189
NZGG (New Zealand Guidelines Group),
    158, 162, 164, 166, 177

odds ratio (OR), 53, 74–6, 189
OTBIBSys, 22, 174, 189
OTDBase, 22, 30–31, 37–8, 174–5, 189
OT process, 5, 9
OTSeeker, 22, 24, 26, 37–8, 67, 106, 108, 121,
    149, 175, 189
outcome measures, 114–20
outcomes, 8, 12–14, 146, 149

p values, 48–52, 190
PEDro, 22, 121, 175, 189
PEDro Rating Scale, 81, 83, 152, 180
phenomenology, 87, 90, 98, 189
PICO, 147
    developing evidence-based questions,
        10–14, 147–8
placebo, 45, 189
probability, 48–50, 189, 190
publication bias, 75, 189
PubMed, 22, 27–8, 37–8, 178, 188–90

qualitative research, 15, 86–104
    appraisal,
        comparison with quantitative
            research, 88
quality assessment, 72, 83, 151–2, 154, 190
quantitative research, 87
    comparison with qualitative research,
        86, 88
questionnaires, 107–108
questions, 9–10, 147–8
    anatomy of, 10–11
    developing evidence-based, 10–11, 147
    examples, 12–14, 148
    well-built, 10–11

randomisation, 45, 56, 190
randomised controlled trial (RCT), 15,
    23–4, 38, 43–66, 87, 106, 147, 188, 190
reflective practice, 128–9
reflexivity, 91, 93–4, 99, 101
relative risk, 53

reliability, 88, 92, 112, 114–18, 120, 190
research, 6
    approaches, 15
    comparison with audit and evidence-
        based practice, 4–5
    definitions, 4
    methodology, 24
    methods,
        utilisation, 138–9
responsiveness, 117–18, 120
rigour, 47–8, 88, 92–5, 190
Rosenthal effect, 63

sampling, 45, 93–4, 96–8, 107–12
ScHARR (School of Health and Related
    Research, 42, 179
search engines, 31, 33
search strategies, 24–5, 38–9, 69–70
    examples, 25–35, 70
searching, 23–39, 148–50
    advanced searches, 33, 35, 38
    examples of searches, 25–35
    hand searching,
        searching the web, 31–5
sensitivity, 117
SIGN (Scottish Intercollegiate Guidelines
    Network), 158, 164, 166, 179
significance,
    clinical, 52–3, 66
    statistical, 48–50, 59, 64, 66, 113, 154, 190
statistical analysis, 48–52, 113, 117
    descriptive statistics, 48–9
    inferential statistics, 49–52
    statistical significance, 48–50, 59, 64, 66,
        113, 154, 190
supervision, 128–9
surveys, 15, 87, 105–14
systematic reviews, 15, 66–85, 106, 145–55,
    188, 190–91

transferability, 93, 94–5, 97, 102, 191
Transtheoretical Model of Change, 140–41,
    143
triangulation, 93–4, 96, 101, 191
trustworthiness, 88, 92–5, 99, 191
type II error, 51

validity, 47, 88, 92, 107, 112, 114, 116, 118,
    120, 191

websites, 31–5, 37–8, 121–5, 175–9
 appraisal, 122–5
 Centre for Evidence-base Medicine
  (CEBM), 176
 evidence-based occupational therapy,
  42
 OTSeeker, 22, 24, 26, 37–8, 67, 106, 108,
  121, 149, 175, 189
 PEDro, 22, 121, 175, 189

PubMed, 22, 27–8, 37–8, 178, 188–90
ScHARR, 42, 179
search engines, 31, 33
 AltaVista, 33
 Excite, 33
 Google, 33, 35, 38, 106
 Google Scholar, 177
 WebCrawler, 33
 Yahoo, 33